Mediterranean Diet for Beginners:

The Complete Guide- 100 Essential Recipes, 30-Day Kick start Meal Plan and the Strategy for Sustainable Weight Loss

By Jerry Allen

Table of Contents

Introduction i

PART 1-Introduction to the Mediterranean Diet and its Health Benefits 2

Chapter 1: Mediterranean In, Garbage Out 1

Chapter 2:It's Allabout a Healthy Discipline, Not Restriction 5

Chapter 3: Mediterranean on a Budget for Both Your Heart and Bank Account 12

PART 2-Health Benefits BeyondThe Heart 20

Chapter 4: Reducing the Risk of Alzheimer's Disease, Diabetes, and Cancer 21

PART 3-Mediterranean Recipes 25

Chapter 5: Rise and Shine! 26
Faster fare 26
For The More Relaxed Morningsandthe Brunch Bunch 40
Easy Lunch Recipes to Get You in Shape 69
Dinner Meals for the Whole Family 111
Vegetarian Dinners for the Mediterranean Diet 154
Easy Mediterranean Desserts 174
Easy Smoothies for Those Busy Days 207

30-Day Meal Plan to Get You Started 215

Introduction

The Mediterranean Diet is one of the best diet plans out there to help you lose weight and feel like the best version of yourself. This diet plan is based on the foods and meals that people in the Mediterranean area like to eat, making it easy to get a ton of variety in your meals. If you have tried out diet plans in the past and they are just not doing the job for you, then it may be time to take a look through this guidebook and get all the information that you need to get started with the Mediterranean diet and finally see some results.

Inside this guidebook, we will take some time to explore the Mediterranean diet and everything that you need to know to make it work for your weight loss goals. We will discuss what the Mediterranean diet is all about, how it can be great for your heart health, other health benefits of this diet plan, and even how to stick with the Mediterranean diet when you are on a budget.

After learning more about this great diet plan and how to get started, this guidebook will move on to some of the best recipes that you can follow. There are some tasty recipes for breakfast, lunch, dinner, and desserts as well as a great 30-day meal plan to help you get started seeing the results in no time.

When you are ready to finally lose weight and feel amazing, make sure to check out this guidebook to help you learn more about the Mediterranean diet today!

PART 1- Introduction to the Mediterranean Diet and its Health Benefits

Chapter 1: Mediterranean In, Garbage Out

Due to the fast and busy lives of people since the recent years, they tend to go to many fastfood chains or any restaurants for a quick bite since they don't have time anymore to cook their own foods at home. They tend to eat processed foods, usually peppered with high levels of sodium, fats, and preservatives that do more harm to the body.

However, it can be observed that many people try to stay away from these kinds of foods and spend less time on this kind of places each day since they now take notice of their lives and the way they're living and wish to leave much longer in a healthier way.

The main reasons are: Some of them have been informed of the many risks that come with habitually eating fast food, *especially the* higher risks of heart problems. Some of them have already started showing visible unwanted weight gain and various other ailments such as having more frequent joint and stomach pains. In addition to those, they have more often than not found themselves feeling more sluggish and tired than they generally should after consuming these "foods". But, correcting and eliminating these problems all begins with being more mindful of what they choose to eat.

At the same time, however, some of those people who *have* now cut and kept out such fare from their culinary repertoires in order to lose weight have given into living by faddish, trendy diets such as Paleo, Ketogenic, and gluten-free, all of which have proven not to be the wisest or healthiest lifestyles to live in the long run.

For example, the Paleo diet is not truly practical for anyone, because while it *does* guarantee weight loss with foods such as nuts, fruit, vegetables, and unprocessed meat, it allows absolutely *no* dairy products, which contain essential nutrients for bone health such as calcium and Vitamin D. Not even those who are lactose intolerant or have other dairy allergies would live an overall healthy life on Paleo because it won't even allow dairy substitutes. Without those nutrients, your kidneys and heart will be more likely to fail.

Also impractical is the Ketogenic (Keto) diet. Any diet that is comprised of high-fat foods and a near-complete lack of fruits and whole grains, both essential for focus and healthy mobility, will not last long because not everyone has the same body type - different amounts of fat take different amounts of time to burn. Plus, eating high-fat foods in copious amounts will result in high cholesterol levels in older age regardless of your body type.

While the gluten-free diet is the most popular of all the three most recent fads, it is also the worst of the three for your health. Unless you *truly* have celiac disease or any other proven gluten-sensitivities, then you should *not* live by the gluten-free diet, because it will actually cause you to *gain* weight, which in turn puts you at a higher risk for heart disease.

Adding to those three fads is another slightly less recent practice of the juice cleanse. That, in addition to the others, will guarantee rapid weight loss in the beginning, but eventually, you'll end up *gaining* back all the lost weight *plus* an additional few extra pounds because you lacked many of the necessary nutrients that weren't allowed in those diets and made up for that by consuming foods very high in fat.

With all that said, we now come down to the real question: Why have people who aim to lose weight and keep their hearts healthy all-around decided to try the Mediterranean diet over any other kind of general eating habit, especially that with a specific name attached to it? For starters, the Mediterranean diet is not really a diet but a lifestyle. Any kind of diet, especially when that term is used in that improper context, really is only a temporary thing, and many quickly lose interest in those since they no longer want to deprive themselves of certain foods and nutrients they love—and need.

Although it's only becoming popular especially amongst Americans, the Mediterranean way of eating is by no means some kind of "trend" or "fad" as many people tend to dismiss it as. It has actually been around for thousands of years and doesn't encourage you to have to "give up" any kinds of foods, so long as you eat them in moderation and balance, which are always the keywords here. You don't have to worry about planning your next "cheat meal" or "cheat day". For example, you want to have a sweet pastry? You can go ahead and have one, as long as this does not become a very habitual thing for you. There is also not one central food that will suddenly make your system all better overnight and keep it that way. If you are really up for this lifestyle, you need to broaden your palate a little, which is one reason choosing your fruits and vegetables by season rather than sticking with one or two types of each fruit and vegetable all year round works best. This also means that you will have more antioxidants such as those that prevent cancer incorporated into your daily life.

Not only will eating Mediterranean help you with your heart and weight loss, it also helps you overcome depression and greatly reduces the risk of diabetes. It also helps to lower your metabolism, which is especially important for the older generation to maintain muscle and bone health. The Mediterranean diet is also preventative in other ways, which will be discussed later on.

While eating Mediterranean is not nearly as restrictive as any fad diet that's ever been created, it still requires you to have certain minor disciplines, all of which will be discussed in more detail in the next chapter. Fair warning: If you are not yet ready to give up any fast-food, processed food or any other "stereotypical" American eating habits, please stop reading this book any further. For those who are truly ready to embark on this new mission: Read on, best of luck, and enjoy!

Chapter 2: It's All about a Healthy Discipline, Not Restriction

When it comes to the Mediterranean diet, there is no limit as to how old you are (although this diet is highly popular amongst the 50-and-older crowd) or what your body type is. It all really depends on how disciplined enough you are to finally give up any kind of processed food and how much more often you're willing to prepare and eat your own meals at home, and preferably, not alone if that's plausible for you.

Don't fret and feel as if you have to completely cut out any food items, carbohydrates or *healthy* fats, such as your omega-3s and omega-9s, so long as you eat each of them in moderation. This lifestyle allows you to utilize all four of the food groups into your habits. It's even vegetarian-friendly, so long as you incorporate fish if you're going to use a protein source that isn't meat. Veganism can also be implemented into this diet, as long as you have the adequate and proper resources.

The Mediterranean diet should be partaken in a social manner. That way, you can focus a bit more on socializing than eating, although you can still take the time to slow down and actually taste and enjoy the food. Generally speaking, the slower pace you eat at, the fuller and more satisfied you feel once you leave the table, without ever having to consume food in such large quantities or even going for second helpings. Eating too fast or too much in front of people is and always has been socially unacceptable, anyway. It has also been proven that those who eat frequently with others while being seated at a table, especially at their own homes or at someone else's, are less likely to develop obesity, heart disease or any other condition that will eventually shorten their lives.

This way of life would still be plausible even if you live alone. There *is* always a time to meal-prep for the week on the weekends, so that you can actually have time to eat a quick breakfast at home before heading out for the day and can even pack a lunch to take with you everyday instead of spending money in the cafeteria (if your workplace has one) or giving into temptation from any nearby fast-food places. It will also be a wise idea to meal-prep if you feel too tired to cook fully when you come home from work. There are meal plans for bachelors and bachelorettes listed later on in this book. Another good idea for those living alone could be to invite friends and family over for meals. If they like, they can also actually prepare and cook the meals *with* you, which can also make for a good time to bond and catch up with them.

As the whole purpose of the Mediterranean diet is to avoid processed foods at all costs, going to a small Gyro joint and ordering a small Mediterranean-style salad with a Gyro does *not* count as an authentic part of this lifestyle. If you have days where you don't feel like cooking and want to eat at a *nice* Italian, Greek or even a French restaurant, that is fine to do as long as you are informed enough about the ingredients in the foods on the menu, as this diet wants you to take it easy on the salt as much as possible.

Another discipline you need to adhere to if you want to truly commit yourself to the Mediterranean diet is the number of types of foods you consume and how careful you are with the quantities of condiments such as olive oil while preparing your meals.

Here are some basics of what you should adhere to if you choose to go on and live this lifestyle:

1.) Cook everything from scratch, and absolutely no processed foods allowed. This includes no beverages with added sugars or artificial sweeteners, no processed meats, and no refined sugars or refined oils.

2.) Butter and margarine are not good for this diet, so you can substitute them both for olive oil. Use it generously, but don't overdo it because while olive oil is a good fat for you, it does have a high caloric content. It's actually better to use olive oil for salad dressing than it is to deep-fry your foods in them. Remember, no more than two tablespoons of olive oil a day. If you're using teaspoons, limit that to 6 or 7 a day. If you're using nuts, you may want to reduce the amount of olive oil you use that day, whether you're using teaspoons *or* tablespoons.

3.) You can get creative and add spices and fresh herbs to your cooking for some extra flavor. Basil, cloves, cumin, fennel, tarragon, garlic, parsley, rosemary, and paprika are just a few of the many spices you could implement into your cooking, and even some herbs can be used just as garnishes.

4.) For your proteins, you *can* have chicken, red meats, and eggs, but all of them should be consumed in moderation. Try to eat fish three times or more each week and add at least one meatless, fully plant-based day a week to your life. The best kinds of fish are fresh and high in omega-3 acids (excellent for your brain), such as herring, trout, sardines, and salmon. Red meat is only good to eat in moderation rather than on a daily basis because habitual red meat-eaters, especially those who eat *processed* red meats, are more likely to have shorter lives. Also, incorporate nuts, your best bet being walnuts, in some of your meals, especially with salads because they are also rich in omega-3 acids. But limit your consumption of nuts to no more than a fourth of a cup a day and make sure they're not candied, roasted, smoked, and keep them lightly salted or unsalted altogether.

5.) Be sure to implement potatoes (preferably sweet or red potatoes if you're not allergic) and other foods rich in fiber and whole grains such as beans, barley, oats, and quinoa into your habits.

6.) Eat dairy every day by supplementing those needs primarily with cheese. Feta and goat cheese works best, but you can use other types of cheese if you don't like either of those.

7.) Eat more vegetables than meats. This is primarily a plant-based diet.

8.) Make sure you choose fresh, seasonal produce, especially when it comes to fruits and vegetables. Be sure to eat at least five servings daily of each for best results. To make sure you're utilizing that, you can start off each meal with a salad and/or a vegetable-based soup, and end them with a piece of fresh fruit.

9.) For dessert each night, opt for a piece of fresh fruit. It is all right to indulge every now and then and have a pastry or piece of cake for dessert as well.

10.) Drink plenty of water. This diet also allows you to have some wine if you like, *with meals,* but no more than six ounces per day. It is recommended that women should drink no more than one glass a day and no more than two glasses daily for men. Beers and hard liquors of any kind, however, are never allowed here.

11.) Don't be afraid of the healthy fats, especially those high in omega-3 and oleic (omega-9) acids. Although fats such as avocado are high in calories, they also help lower cholesterol levels, so enjoy the avocado! Eating foods that contain healthy fats do *not* contribute to weight gain.

12.) Controlling portions on your plate should be more of a focus than counting the calories or carbs. The best way to know that your portions are controlled is to set up your plates according to the Harvard Ratio:

- ½ a plate of veggies, as this is a primarily plant-based diet. Artichokes, broccoli, turnips, cucumbers, kale, lettuce, okra, peas, pumpkin, potatoes (as long as they are not deep-fried), and radishes are good examples of veggies if you're not sure what to get, so long as they're in tune to whatever season it is. For example, you might not want to eat cucumbers in the winter.

- ¼ a plate of whole grains such as whole wheat pasta, brown rice, oats, quinoa, and barley. Stay away from white rice and white bread because they release energy too quickly and won't leave you as satiated.

- ¼ a plate of protein. You can eat red meat every once in a while, but your main sources of protein should be beans, chicken or fishes.

NOTE: Not only is portion control important, but the *size* of your plate is, too. The larger the plate size, the more likely the purpose of portion control will be defeated.

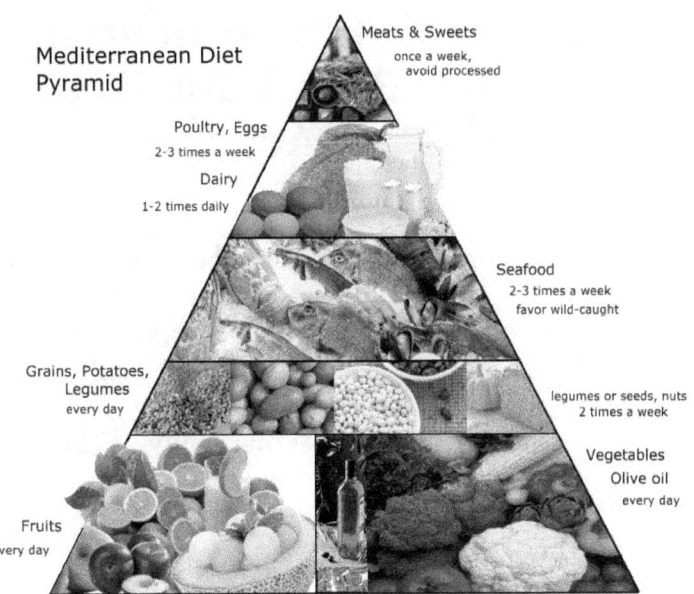

Fresh Fruits & Vegetables: Every day, every meal, 1/2 cup cooked, 1 cup raw

Chapter 3: Mediterranean on a Budget for Both Your Heart and Bank Account

Many people are skeptical about adopting the Mediterranean culinary lifestyle because they fear that they will be unable to afford the food items and ingredients needed to accommodate it daily. Many also fear not being able to live a healthy lifestyle in general because of finances. While many of the foods used as part of the Mediterranean diet are organic, there's no law that says they *have* to be, even though organic products in some stores have become more affordable and accessible.

But, there *are* quite a few ways to be able to live this lifestyle without having to shell out large amounts of money at the grocery store and/or the farmer's market.

1. Utilize canned beans

    Canned beans are almost always on sale at major chain supermarkets and sometimes, even at farmer's market-style establishments. Full of proteins and fibers, you don't even have to make a fuss while making them. You can even use these on your salads or make chili with them. You can also use this as a dip for veggies and healthy, whole-grain chips.

2. VediVidi Veggies!

Another reason why it is stressed that more veggies than meat should be consumed is that the indigenous Mediterranean (from Greece, Italy, and Southern France) lived during a time when meat was considered a luxury. Stocking up on more meat than veggies actually saves so much more on your grocery bill per year than loading up on meats.

3. Eggs are not just for breakfast.

    Eggs are often on sale and affordable. You can also make frittatas with cherry tomatoes and spinach and cheeses for both lunch and dinner. Frittatas are filling and they don't take that long to prepare. Some people also take to frying eggs and using them as sandwich toppings. You can never go wrong with an egg-and-cheese sandwich on whole grain bread or a whole grain pita. Or, if you're adventurous enough, an egg on top of a quinoa burger patty would be good for lunch or dinner.

4. Go to the farmer's market late in the day.

    If you want to go to the farmer's market to get your foods needed, your best bet is to go later on in the day, particularly right before closing time, because much of the produce there is cheaper, as the farmers would rather sell them than pack them up for the next day.

5. If your town has a local community supported agriculture group, join it.

At community-supported agricultures or CSAs, their produce is even cheaper than the produce you'll find at the grocery stores. All produce is local at CSAs, and you, in turn, will be helping support local farmers and grocers.

6. Rather than your traditional pasta sauce, make puttanesca.

Puttanesca is a type of pasta "sauce" whose ingredients include tomatoes, garlic, and anchovies. All of these ingredients are very affordable and can be used multiple times for your pasta dishes.

7. Sales mean stocking, stocking, stocking

If there is a sale at your grocery store, especially on seafood, eggs, spices (preferably in bulk to save money), vegetables (frozen, fresh or canned will work), fruits, herbs, pasta, grains such as beans, rice, lentils, oats, and barley (all preferably in bulk as well) and nuts, be sure to stock up as much as possible. You can even freeze many of these ingredients to save for later and to make them last longer. At the same time, don't wait until the last minute, meaning waiting until it's close to the expiration date, to use all these foods and ingredients. Doing this will make for many modest yet inventive, hearty, delicious meals. Not only will you be saving your money, you'll also be saving time, and what better way to utilize some of that saved time by using some of the ingredients to make your own stock, such as chicken broth? Later on, I will include some

Mediterranean meals to make when you're on a budget and/or living alone.

8. Food-freezing fundamentals

Here are some specific freezing methods to use for each kind of food, and how long they can be stored for:

MEATS AND SEAFOODS

Divide the meats and seafood accordingly, depending on how much you normally eat in one sitting and wrap it as tightly as possible with freezer paper.

Recommended storage time:

- 4-12 months (steaks and chops)
- 3-4 months (ground)
- 9-12 months (poultry)
- 6 months (lean fish, e.g. cod and tilapia)
- 2-3 months (fatty fish, e.g. salmon)
- 3-6 months (shellfish)
- 10 months (shrimp)

NUTS

Place the nuts into a sealable bag, then label and date.

Recommended storage time: 6-12 months

HERBS

Wash the herbs and let them dry. Then put them in a freezer bag and press out all the air.

Recommended storage time: 1-3 years

BERRIES

Wash and drain fresh berries, before pouring them onto a baking sheet. Make sure that they are in one nice layer to prevent clumping. Place the berries into the freezer until they are all frozen. Then transfer the frozen berries into a sealable bag with all the air out, and then put into the freezer until you need them.

Recommended storage time: 10 months

CHEESES

Wrap the cheeses very tightly with freezer paper, then label and date.

Recommended storage time: 6 months, for both hard and soft cheeses.

TIPS

- Make sure your freezer is always at a temperature of 0 degrees or lower. Keeping it at those temperatures prevents bacteria and other unwanted microbes from getting into the food.

- Eliminate as much air exposure as possible to prevent freezer burn.

9. Hydrate, hydrate, hydrate!

As this diet strongly suggests you drink plenty of water, you can save money, as well as the environment, by investing in a water filter for your kitchen faucet at home rather than buying jugs and bottles of water all the time. This diet also doesn't allow you to drink any beverages with added sugars or artificial sweeteners, so if you want something other than water, you could always have tea, from the bags or sachets, that is. If you don't want to drink your tea hot. You can steep it into a mug or thermos filled with ice cubes. If you want to sweeten your tea or just give it a little extra kick, do so with honey (preferably locally made honey from the farmer's market) or squeeze a little lemon into it. For your morning coffee, you can drink it just black or add some low-fat creamer if you want flavor.

Another thing to keep in mind is that maintaining this diet is by absolutely *no* means a substitute for physical exercise. As a matter of fact, it is recommended that you perform some sort of exercise on a *daily* basis because both the Mediterranean diet and exercise are keys to a longer life. You can consume a whole plethora of fruits and vegetables and drink gallons of water each day, but the truth is still this: Without enough and adequate physical exercise, your joints will stiffen, your metabolism will be higher than normal, and your heart will have to work harder to make up for the lack of exercise. The good thing, though, is that your daily exercise needs don't have to be costly such as a gym membership that you might only end up using twice a week. You can start by doing some walking before you head off to work each day if time allows. If you can't do that, exercises even as simple as stretching/yoga and a few sit-ups will keep you both physically and mentally sound. It is shown that exercise can also help curb your appetite.

With all the time you saved by stocking up on sale foods, buying in bulk, and prepping your meals for the week, you can also make a day of calling up a friend to go exercising with. Not only should you encourage each other's healthy habits by eating together, but also plan activities to do together such as bike riding, running, hiking, swimming, and others that are especially heart-healthy. Or, you can even still do all of these alone if your friends can't make it that day.

With all of this, you should also make sure you always leave yourself enough time for leisure and adequate rest.

PART 2-Health Benefits Beyond The Heart

Chapter 4: Reducing the Risk of Alzheimer's Disease, Diabetes, and Cancer

The Mediterranean diet is not only about preserving your heart and bones but also your brain, as it is needed to stay healthy in order to enable mindful eating, from the foods you choose to its specific portions. While it is still unknown whether or not this diet *definitely* will reduce your risk of developing Alzheimer's and/or dementia, there are some beliefs that lead to that possibility. One of them is that it can reduce brain tissue loss, something that comes along with Alzheimer's. It might also help reduce the risk of cognitive impairments, many of which progress into Alzheimer's. Other studies show that eating lots of fruits and veggies, both high in antioxidants, can protect the brain cells from damages that cause Alzheimer's and dementia. The more a person sticks with this style of eating, the lower they risk losing memory and developing this disease. It also helps keep cholesterol under control, which in turn will reduce the risk of memory loss. Other essential foods preventative of Alzheimer's are: leafy green veggies, a salad in addition to one other vegetable each day, fruits specifically in the berry family at least twice a week (although non-berry fruits are allowed as well), beans, three servings of whole grains daily, fish at least once a week to protect your brain function, and at least two poultry servings a week. Olive oil helps retain your cognitive skills. You can also have up to *one* glass of wine per day. But stay away from butter, margarine, and fried foods, and limit your sweet/pastry intake to no more than five per week.

Those who make the Mediterranean diet a consistent part of their lives rather than a fleeting thing will be sure to have their sugar under control. This diet allows sugar but not refined or artificial, and that discipline greatly lowers the risk of type 2 diabetes. However, those who already are type 2 diabetic, can use this as a way to lower cholesterol and keep their blood sugar levels under control at all times, in addition to enabling weight loss. However, some diabetics who make the Mediterranean diet their way of life are still required to take diabetes medication to control their blood sugar, mainly because their diets allow for no more than 30% of healthy fats per day and that they're not eating enough whole grains, fruits or vegetables per day.

It has also been proven that with less meat, especially *red* meats, your risk of getting cancer will be reduced by up to 50%. To achieve the best results, be sure to swap out meat at least 2-3 times a week for fish, eggs, seeds, grains (quinoa is a great source for this), and nuts (particularly walnuts or pistachios).

There is also a possible correlation between the reduction of breast cancer risk and the Mediterranean diet. Refraining from alcoholic beverage intake, save for a maximum of a glass of wine a day, has been known to reduce the chances of having breast cancer, particularly in women over 50, as has the regular consumption of leafy green vegetables such as kale, parsley, spinach, and lettuce. Other than that, no direct correlation between the diet and reducing the risk has yet been found.

This way of life is also beneficial for your colon and rectum. If you incorporate more fish and fruit, in addition to your vegetables and whole grains, into your eating habits, then your risk of colorectal cancer is reduced. Generally speaking, the more foods suitable for this diet that you consume, the better off you are, especially when you go for your colonoscopy to see if there are any cancer-causing polyps developing in your system.

In addition to helping your body fight against those diseases, this diet helps prevent any future eyesight problems and failures, especially if your diet consists of kale, which contains a powerful antioxidant for your eyesight called lutein. Fatty acids found in most fish keep the muscles, cells, organs, and nerves functioning properly so that your heart beats at a regular rate and that your blood pressure stays under control.

Now that you have a general idea of what foods to purchase and the right disciplines and life choices *beyond* food to make and keep the Mediterranean diet a part of your everyday life, as well as very specific instructions on how to save money and retain the freshness of your foods and ingredients, you are now ready to have a look at some breakfast, lunch, dinner, simple salad, snack, and even some vegan-friendly recipes. I will also include beverages such as smoothies and juice recipes good for the Med diet.

PART 3- Mediterranean Recipes

Chapter 5:
Rise and Shine!

This chapter will feature recipes for quick breakfasts for your workaday mornings, more leisurely breakfasts, and even some brunch ideas to share with friends and/or family.

Faster fare

Note: Some of the recipes featured in this breakfast chapter can also be used for lunch, especially if you're not eating lunch at home.

Mediterranean scrambled eggs with spinach, tomato, and feta

Cooking Time: 4 mins
Preparation time: 2 mins

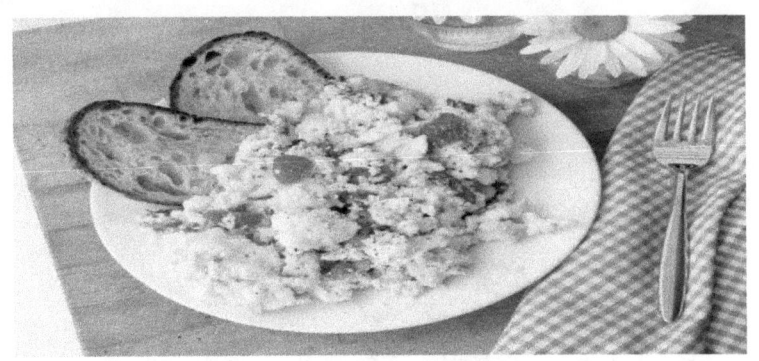

Ingredients:

- Vegetable oil (1 Tbsp.)
- Tomatoes, diced (.33 c.)
- 1 cup of baby spinach
- 2 tbsp. of cubed Feta cheese
- 3 eggs
- Salt and pepper if you want taste

Directions:
1. Place a skillet onto the stove and let the oil heat up.
2. Sautéyour tomatoes and spinach until the leaves of the spinach wilts.
3. Add the scrambled eggs into the skillet, mixing them with the spinach and tomatoes.
4. 30 seconds later, add the Feta cheese.
5. Cook until the egg is cooked the way that you like them. Season a bit before serving.

Mediterranean Egg Salad

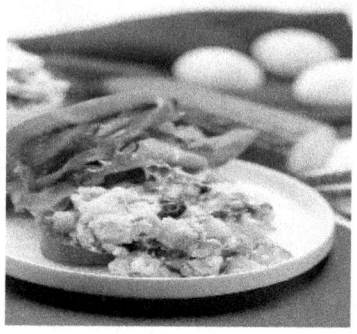

This can be eaten alone or on a sandwich and works either as a breakfast or lunch item.

Ingredients:

- 8 large hardboiled eggs, chopped (best to hard-boil your eggs the night before if you want this for breakfast)
- ½ cup red onion, finely chopped
- ¼ cup chopped olives
- ½ cup chopped cucumber
- ½ cup chopped sundried tomatoes, make sure any and all excess oil is drained *before* you chop them.
- Freshly ground black pepper, if you want taste
- ½ cup plain Greek yogurt
- 1 ½ tsp. oregano
- ¼ tsp. cumin
- ½ tsp. sea salt
- A splash of lemon juice

Directions:

1. Place in a bowl the hardboiled eggs.
2. Add your tomatoes, olives, onions, and cucumber.
3. Then add the cumin, lemon juice, Greek yogurt, pepper, salt, and mix everything together.

This has a shelf-life of up to one week in the fridge.

Sunny Greek Quinoa Breakfast Bowl

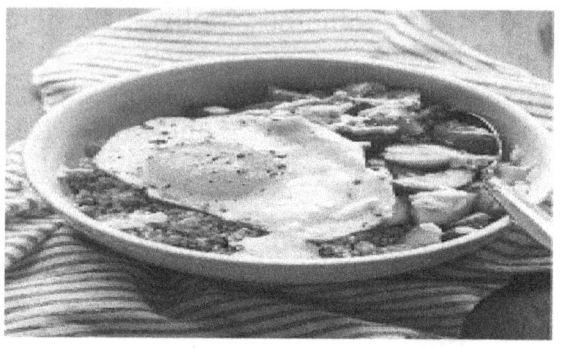

Total time: 10 mins

Ingredients:

- ¼ cup quinoa
- ¼ cup water
- ¼ cup almond milk
- 1/4 cup sliced cucumber
- 2 tbsp Tzatziki sauce
- ¼ tsp. coconut oil
- ½ cup sliced cherry tomatoes
- 1 egg, sunny-side up
- 1 c plain Greek yogurt

Directions:

1. Combine quinoa, water, and milk into a saucepan and boil.
2. In about 4 minutes, lower the heat and simmer until all the liquid has been absorbed. This process takes 8 minutes.
3. Place this mixture, topped with the tomato and cucumber, into a small bowl.

4. Prepare another small bowl to break the egg. Over medium heat, heat up a coconut oil on a non-stick pan. When the oil melts, gently slide the egg into a pan.
5. Cook the egg for 2-3 minutes, and then add a dash of salt and pepper.
6. Gently slide the egg on top of quinoa mixture, and drizzle with Tzatziki sauce.

Honey-Caramelized Figs with Yogurt

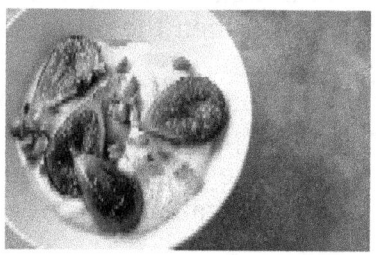

Total time: 10 mins

Ingredients:

- 1 tbsp. honey
- 2 cups of plain, low-fat Greek yogurt
- 8 oz. of fresh figs, all cut in half
- A pinch of ground cinnamon
- ¼ cup chopped pistachios

Directions:

1. Over medium heat, heat honey in skillet.
2. With the sides down, cook figs for about 5 minutes until they're caramelized.
3. Serve figs over yogurt and cinnamon.

Mediterranean Toast

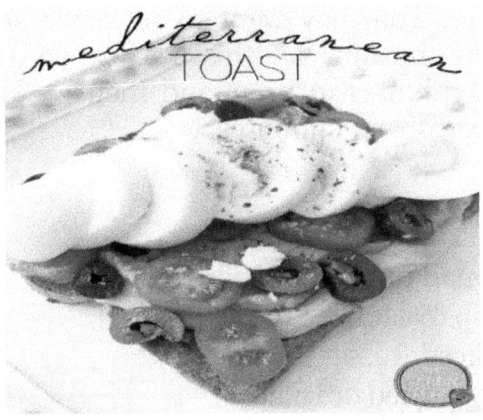

Ingredients:

- 1 slice of whole wheat or multigrain toast
- ¼ mashed avocado
- 1 tbsp. roasted red pepper hummus
- 3 sliced Greek olives
- 3 sliced cherry or grape tomatoes
- 1 sliced hard-boiled egg
- 1 ½ tsp. of reduced fat crumbled Feta cheese

Directions:

1. Toast the bread and spread it with the hummus and avocado.
2. Add the tomatoes and olives.
3. Add the sliced hard-boiled egg and season it with salt and pepper.

Mediterranean Potato Hash

Note: You may want to set aside some extra time in the morning for this because you may need about ten minutes to prep, and then cooking it will consume another 14 minutes.

Ingredients:

- 1 small finely chopped red onion
- 1 tsp. Za'atar
- 2 diced Russet potatoes
- 1 tsp. dried oregano
- 2 chopped garlic cloves
- 1 cup of rinsed and dried canned chickpeas
- 1 ½ tsp. ground allspice
- 1 ½ tbsp. olive oil
- 4 poached eggs
- 2 chopped Roma tomatoes
- 1 cup of chopped fresh parsley, no stems
- 1 small chopped yellow onion
- 1 tsp. white vinegar
- A pinch of sugar
- 1 tsp. paprika, sweet or smoked
- 1 lb. asparagus, ends removed, chopped into ¼ inch pieces
- 1 tsp. coriander
- ½ cup crumbled Feta cheese
- 1 tsp. dried oregano

Directions:

1. Take out a skillet and add some olive oil into it. When the oil hot, add the potatoes, garlic, and onion. Season these and let them cook to make the potatoes tender.
2. When the potatoes are soft, add in the spices, asparagus, and chickpeas. Stir together. Lower the heat after another 5 minutes to keep everything warm.
3. Bring out another pot and let some water simmer in it. When the water is simmering, break a few eggs into a bowl and add some water.
4. Cook for a few minutes and then take the eggs out. Make sure to drain off the water.
5. Take your potato mixture from the heat before adding the Feta cheese, red onions, parsley, and tomatoes. Put the eggs on top and serve.

Mediterranean Breakfast Egg Muffins

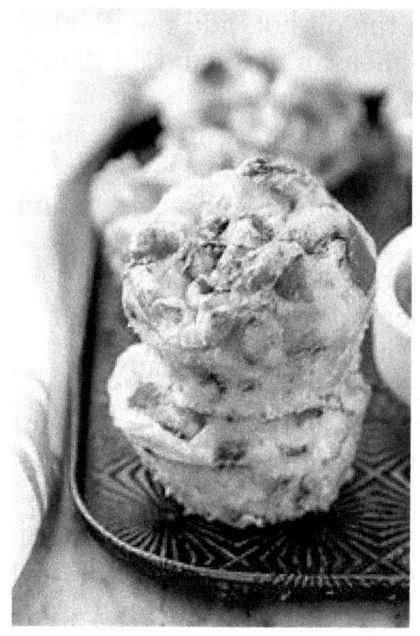

Ingredients:

- 3 large eggs
- Cooking oil spray
- 25g low-fat grated cheddar cheese
- Salt and pepper
- ¼ finely chopped red pepper
- 2 tbsp. skim milk
- 25g finely chopped baby spinach
- 35g finely chopped leek
- 4 tbsp. grated Parmesan cheese
- 1 chopped tomato, deseeded

Directions:

1. Turn on the oven and give it time to heat up to 375 degrees. Prepare a muffin tin with a little bit of cooking spray.
2. In a jug, whisk milk, parmesan cheese, and eggs and season the mixture with pepper and salt.
3. Equally divide the mixture into the six compartments of the muffin tin.
4. Sprinkle the grated cheese evenly amongst the six muffins.
5. Bake until the oven is set for about 15-20 minutes.

Mediterranean Breakfast Tostadas

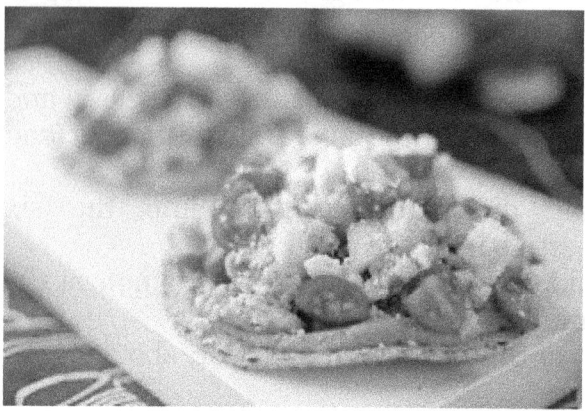

Cooking Time: 5 mins
Prep time: 10 mins

Ingredients:

- 4 tostadas
- 1/2 cup skim milk
- 8 beaten eggs
- ½ tsp. oregano
- ½ tsp. garlic powder
- ½ chopped and seeded cucumber
- ¼ cup crumbled Feta
- ½ chopped green onions
- ½ cup diced tomatoes
- ½ cup diced red pepper
- ½ cup roasted red pepper hummus

Directions:

1. Cook for about 3 minutes the red peppers in a skillet on medium heat.

2. Add garlic powder, milk, eggs, onions, and oregano, stirring for about 2 minutes.
3. Put the egg mixture, cucumber, tomatoes, hummus, and Feta cheese. These should be eaten immediately.

For The More Relaxed Mornings and the Brunch Bunch

Shakshouka Classic Mediterranean Breakfast

Cooking Time: 20 mins
Prep time: 10 mins

Ingredients:

- Salt and pepper for taste
- 1 finely sliced onion
- 2 finely sliced red bell peppers
- 2Garlic cloves, chopped
- 1 15oz. chopped tomato
- ½ tsp. of spicy harissa
- 1 tsp. of sugar
- 4 eggs
- 1 tsp. of sugar
- 1 tbsp. of chopped parsley
- Olive oil (1 tsp.)

Directions:

1. Bring out a skillet and heat it up nice and warm on your stove. Add in the prepared peppers and onions, and season with some garlic.
2. These need to cook together until warm. Then add in the tomatoes and harissa.
3. After another seven minutes, add salt and pepper for seasoning.

4. Make 4 indentations into each pepper with a wooden spoon and place the egg in each indentation.
5. Cover skillet and let the ingredients cook together until the eggs are all done.
6. Sprinkle parsley onto it and serve with pita bread or crusty bread.

Veggie Mediterranean Quiche

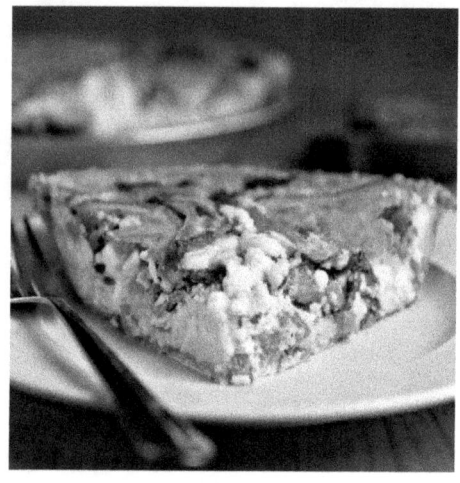

Cooking Time: 55 mins
Prep time: 15 mins

Ingredients:

- ½ cup sundried tomatoes
- 1 diced red pepper
- 2Garlic cloves
- 1 homemade pie crust
- 1 tsp. dried oregano
- 1 diced onion
- ¼ cup sliced Kalamata olives
- 2 c. Spinach
- 1 ¼ cup of milk
- 4 large eggs
- 2 Tbsp Olive oil
- 1 tsp. dried parsley
- 1/3 cup crumbled Feta cheese
- 1 cup divided shredded cheese

Directions:
1. Take out a measuring cup and add your tomatoes inside. Boil some water in a small pot and then pour the tomatoes inside. After a few minutes, take the tomatoes out of the water, drain them, and chop into smaller pieces.
2. Turn on the oven and give it time to heat up to 375 degrees. Bring out a pie plate for this recipe.
3. Cook the garlic and onion for a couple of minutes on a skillet with a hot olive oil. Then add in the parsley, olives, spinach, and oregano.
4. After five more minutes, take the skillet from the heat. This is when you can stir in the Feta cheese and tomatoes.
5. Scoop the mixture into the pie crust and spread it evenly all over.
6. Whisk together the eggs, salt, pepper, ½ a cup of cheddar cheese and milk.
7. Evenly pour that mixture onto the spinach mixture. Add on some more cheese to the top of it all.
8. Time the over for 50 minutes and bake the mixture in the oven.
9. Take it out of the oven afterward and cool for 10-15 minutes.

Mediterranean Omelette

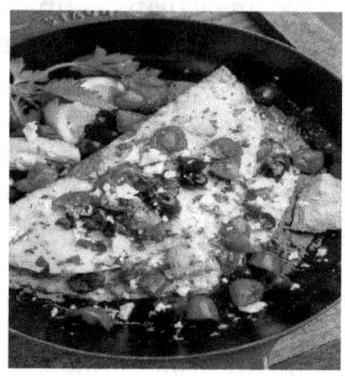

Prep time: 5 mins
Cooking Time: 10 mins

Ingredients:

- Eggs (2)
- Milk (1 tsp.)
- 1 tsp. olive oil
- 2 tbsp. diced tomato
- 1 artichoke heart, cut into quarters
- 1 tbsp. crumbled Feta cheese
- 2 tbsp. sliced Kalamata olives
- 1 tbsp romesco sauce
- Salt, pepper, and oregano for taste.

Directions:

1. Let the oil heat up in a skillet and pour in the mixture of egg, oregano, milk, salt, and pepper.

2. Before you add the Feta, artichoke, tomatoes, and olives per half of the egg, make sure the egg is cooked enough to where it's set.
3. Cook the eggs until set, remove them from heat, and top it with romesco sauce.

Mediterranean Breakfast Salad

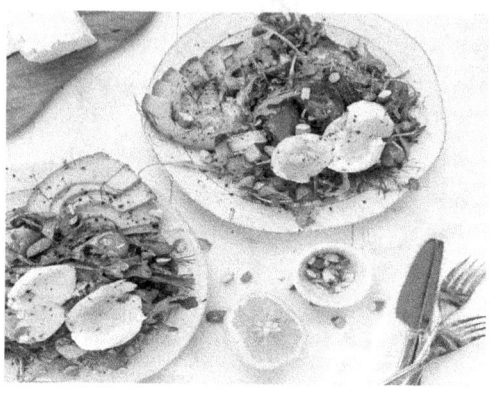

Ingredients:

- 4 eggs
- 2 c. Cherry tomatoes
- 1 lemon
- 10 cups arugula
- ½ unseeded, chopped cucumber
- 1 cup chopped whole natural almonds
- ½ cup chopped mixed herbs (use any kinds of herbs, but mint and dill work best for this)
- 1 large avocado
- Olive oil
- 1 cup cooked quinoa

Directions:

1. Fill up a pot with some boiling water. When the water is bubbling, add in the eggs and let it simmer. Let them cook for a bit.
2. After six minutes, take the eggs out of the pot and put them in some cold water. Peel the shells off after they have cooled down.

3. Combine tomatoes, arugula, quinoa, and cucumbers into a bowl. Add a bit of pepper, olive oil, and salt to this and toss the salad a bit.
4. Top the salad with avocado and sliced egg, and then sprinkle it with almonds and herbs. Season the salad how you wish and add a bit of lemon to the mix as well.

Greek-Style Frittata

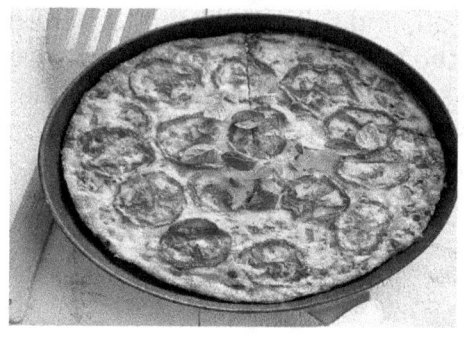

Cooking Time: 10 mins
Prep time: 15 mins

Ingredients:

- 1 tsp. dried oregano
- .5 c. Chopped roasted sweet red peppers
- ½ cup boiling water
- ½ cup of dried tomato slices
- .25 c. Reduced-fat crumbled Feta cheese
- 1/3 cup Italian olive antipasto, marinated in garlic and herbs
- Eggs (8)
- 1 tbsp. Olive oil
- Pepper

Directions:

1. Turn on the oven and let it heat up to 425 degrees. Combine the dried tomatoes together with your water and let them mix together in the bowl for a bit. Then drain the tomatoes, setting aside the liquid.

2. Whisk the eggs well in a large bowl. Stir in cheese, peppers, and oregano. Lightly drain and chop the antipasto and stir it, along with the tomato liquid you have set aside, into egg mixture.
3. On medium heat, heat olive oil into a skillet and pour the egg mixture into it, topped with the dried tomatoes. Bake the skillet with this mixture for 10-13 minutes.
4. Sprinkle with pepper and fresh oregano (optional)

Kale and Goat Cheese Frittata

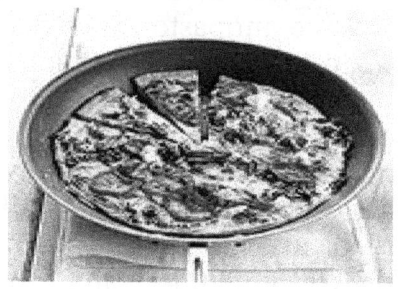

Total time: 25 mins

Ingredients:

- ¼ cup thinly-sliced dried tomatoes 4 egg whites
- 6 eggs
- ¼ tsp. salt
- 1 oz. crumbled goat cheese
- 1Sliced onion
- 2 tsp. Olive oil
- 1/8 tsp. ground pepper
- 2 cups of coarsely and freshly torn kale

Directions:

1. Preheat broiler. Bring out your skillet and heat up the oil until it is smoking. Cook the kale and onion in the oil for a bit.
2. At the same time, whisk the pepper, salt, eggs, and the egg whites together until smooth. After ten minutes have passed, pour this over your kale.

3. Lower the heat a bit and let it cook. Check on the egg mixture to see if it is about to set or not.
4. When the egg is set, sprinkle on the tomatoes and goat cheese.
5. Place the whole skillet in the broiler and let it cook for a few more minutes.
6. Cool the frittata down before slicing into wedges and serving.

Greek Vegetable and Feta Cheese Pie

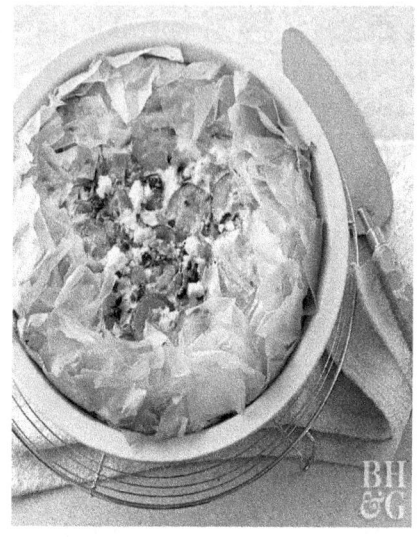

Cooking Time: 40 mins
Prep time: 35 mins

Ingredients:

- ¼ tsp. salt
- 10 sheets Phyllo dough
- 1/8 tsp. ground nutmeg
- 1 cup of large chopped onion
- ½ cups of thinly sliced medium zucchini
- 1 Tbsp. Olive oil
- 10 oz. Chopped spinach
- 2 Eggs
- 1 ½ cups of evaporated low-fat milk
- ¾ cup of chopped medium sweet red pepper
- ¼ tsp. freshly ground pepper
- 2 cloves of minced garlic

- 2oz of reduced fat crumbled Feta cheese

Directions:

1. Turn on the oven and let it heat up to 375 degrees. Add some oil to a skillet before cooking the pepper and onion. Then add zucchini and cook for 4 minutes or until it browns. Add garlic, spinach and 1 tsp. of salt, and cook for 2 minutes.
2. Combine eggs, milk, 1 tsp. of salt, ground pepper, and nutmeg into a bowl.
3. Prepare your pie plate and then add some of the dough into it. Gently press the sheet into the bottom and sides of the pie plate. Repeat this step with the rest of the phyllo sheets and place them all in a crisscross pattern.
4. Evenly spread vegetable mixture over the phyllo and sprinkle with cheese. Pour the egg mixture over this. Fold all the overlapping ends of phyllo towards the middle of pie plate. Spray cooking spray over phyllo, and gently press to keep its shape.
5. Bake it in the oven for 40 minutes. Once done, cool for a while. Slice up the pie and serve.

Mediterranean Breakfast Sandwiches

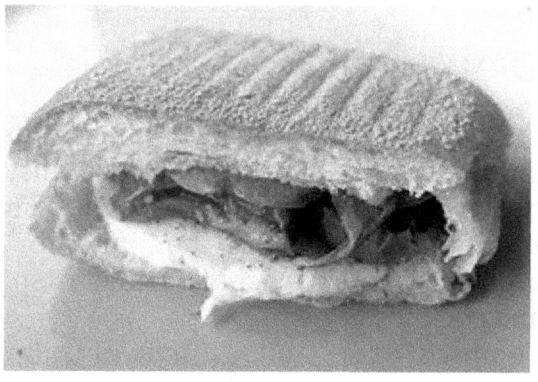

Total time to make: 20 mins

Ingredients:

- 4 multigrain sandwich thins
- ½ tbsp. of crushed dried rosemary or 1 tbsp. of snipped fresh rosemary
- 4 tsp. of olive oil
- 4 Eggs
- 2 c. Spinach leaves
- 1 medium tomato, thinly cut into 8 slices
- 1/8 tsp. Kosher salt
- 4 tbsp. reduced-fat Feta cheese
- Pepper

Directions:

1. Turn on the oven and let it heat up to 375 degrees. Take the cut ends of bread and brush with some oil. Put them onto your baking sheet and heat up in the oven for a bit.

2. Take out your skillet and heat up the rosemary and the oil. Break an egg onto the skillet and cook for a bit. Use your spatula so that you can break the eggs, flipping around halfway through to make sure the eggs are done.
3. Place each bottom halves of sandwich thins onto 4 plates. Top with the tomato, eggs, some cheese, and spinach. Season and serve.

Fava Beans with Pita Bread

Cooking Time: 15 mins
Prep time: 10 mins

Ingredients:

- 1 ½ tbsp. of olive oil
- 1 tsp. ground cumin
- 1 crushed garlic clove
- 1 15oz can of undrained Fava beans
- .25 c. Chopped parsley
- ¼ cup lemon juice
- 1 Onion, chopped
- 4 whole grain pita bread pockets
- 1 Tomato
- seasonings

Directions:

1. On a non-stick pan, heat the olive oil.
2. Cook the onion, garlic, and tomato to the skillet. Then add in the fava beans and the liquids that come with them. Bring to a boil.
3. Add parsley, cumin, and lemon juice and heat them on medium for five minutes. Season with the pepper, salt, and pepper flakes.
4. In another skillet, add in your pita bread and warm them up before using.
5. The pita can be served either on the side or mixed in with the beans.

Yogurt and Honey Fruit Delight

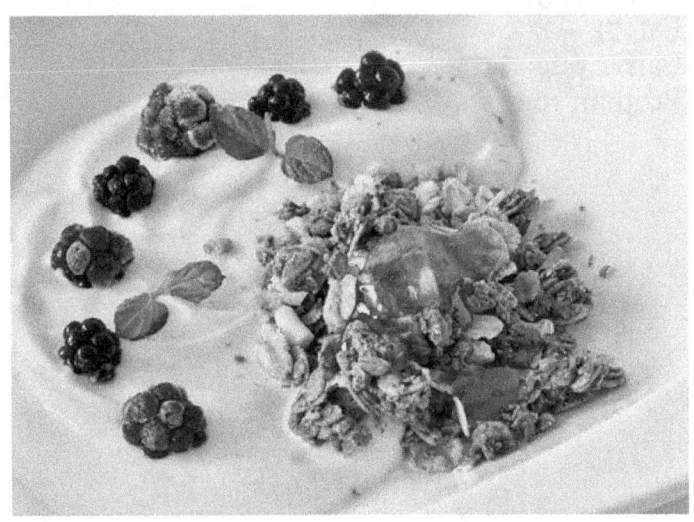

Cooking Time: 0 min
Prep Time: 10 Mins

Ingredients:

- Sunflower and pumpkin seeds (.5 c.)
- Raspberries (1 pint)
- Honey (.5 c.)
- Greek yogurt, plain (4 c.)

Directions:

1. Divide up the yogurt between a few serving dishes.
2. Drizzle with honey, using as much as you would like, and then add some raspberries.

Nutritional Information:

Calories: 377
Fat: 7g
Carbs: 62g
Protein: 16g

Apricot Muesli

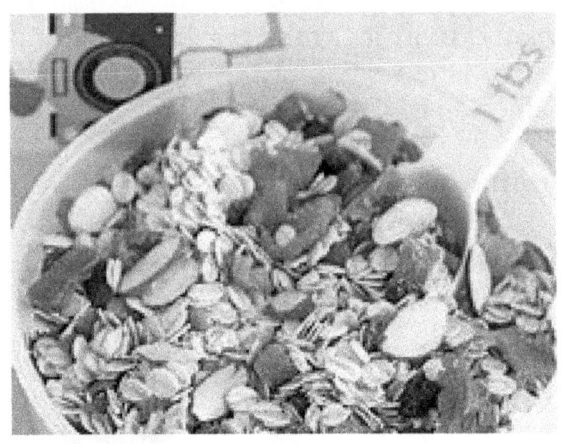

Cooking Time: 0 min
Prep Time: 15 mins

Ingredients:

- Cinnamon (1 tsp.)
- Lemon zest (1 Tbsp.)
- Honey (.25 c.)
- Chopped apricots (.5 c.)
- Almond milk (1.5 c.)
- Chopped pistachios (.25 c.)
- Rolled barley (2 c.)

Directions:

1. Take out a bowl and then stir in the cinnamon, lemon zest, honey, apricots, almond milk, and grains.

2. Cover up the bowl and let it set in the fridge overnight.
3. In the morning, take the bowl out and divide the mixture between four bowls before serving with pistachios on top.

Nutritional Information:

> Calories: 371
> Fat: 3g
> Carbs; 54g
> Protein: 8g

Breakfast Polenta

Cooking Time: 10 mins
Prep Time: 10 mins

Ingredients:

- 1.75 c. Instant polenta
- 2 tsp.Salt
- 4 Tbsp Olive oil
- 6 c.Water

Directions:

1. Place your liquid into a big soup pot and then let it heat up to bubbling. Add in the salt and then whisk the polenta in as well.
2. Let this cook on a medium heat until the polenta becomes thick and you notice that the grain is tender.
3. Stir in the olive oil. Ladle this into bowls before serving.

Nutritional Information:

Calories: 172
Fat: 15g
Carbs: 10g
Protein: 1g

Zucchini Muffins

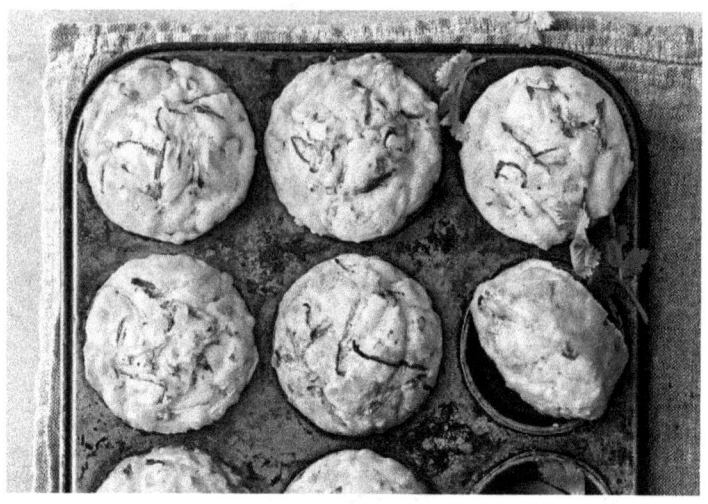

Cooking Time: 20 mins
Prep Time: 15 mins

Ingredients:

- Baking powder (2 tsp.)
- Orange zest (1 Tbsp.)
- Chopped walnuts (.5 c.)
- Salt
- Baking soda (1 tsp.)
- Shredded zucchini (1.5 c.)
- Almond flour (1 c.)
- Vanilla (1 tsp.)
- Olive oil (3 Tbsp.)
- Honey (.25 c.)
- Cinnamon (1 tsp.)

- Eggs (2)
- Whole wheat flour (1 c.)

Directions:

1. Turn on your oven and give it time to heat up to 375 degrees. Spray a cooking spray to your prepared muffin pan.
2. Mix together the eggs, olive oil, zucchini, and honey, and stir them together well.
3. Then add in the baking powder, almond flour, wheat flour, vanilla, orange zest, salt, cinnamon, and baking soda. Fold in your walnuts.
4. Scoop this batter into your muffin tin and place it into the oven.
5. After 20 minutes, the muffins should be done. Take the muffins out and allow them time to cool down before serving.

Nutritional Information:

Calories: 163
Fat: 9g
Carbs: 17g
Protein: 2g

Baked Eggs

Cooking Time: 10 mins
Prep Time: 10 mins

Ingredients:

- Pepper
- Salt
- Parmesan cheese (.5 c.)
- Eggs (8)
- Olive oil (4 tsp.)

Directions:

1. Turn on the oven and let it heat up to 400 degrees. Place a bit of oil inside four ramekins.
2. Break two of your eggs into each ramekin and divide the cheese on top. Season with some pepper and salt.
3. Bake the eggs for ten minutes. Serve.

Nutritional Information:

Calories: 212
Fat: 17g
Carbs: 1g
Protein: 16g

Feta Frittata

Cooking Time: 25 mins
Prep Time: 15 mins

Ingredients:

- Feta cheese (2 oz.)
- Beaten eggs (12)
- Dried oregano (1 tsp.)
- Chopped olives (.25 c.)
- Chopped red peppers, roasted (.25 c.)
- Salt
- Pepper
- Chopped chard (1 bunch)
- Olive oil (1 Tbsp.)

Directions:

1. Prepare a pie plate coated with some oil. Also, heat up the oven to 375 degrees.
2. Add the pepper, salt, and chard to the pie plate and then put it all in the oven. After 10 minutes, take this out of the oven and sprinkle the oregano, olives, and red pepper on top.
3. Slowly pour your eggs into the pie plate and top with the feta cheese. Put the pie plate back in the oven to warm up.
4. After 25 minutes, you should check to see if the eggs are set. If they are, you can remove this from the oven and slice it up before serving.

Nutritional Information:

Calories: 184
Fat: 14g
Carbs: 3g
Protein: 13g

Batsaria (Spanakopita withoutthe Phyllo)

Cooking Time: 55 mins
Prep time: 25 mins

Ingredients:

For spinach mixture:

- 2 tbsp. olive oil
- 4 cloves of peeled and finely chopped garlic
- 1 pinch freshly ground pepper
- 2 1-lb. bags of fresh baby spinach
- 1 small finely chopped yellow onion
- ½ Feta cheese
- 4 eggs
- 1 bunch chopped scallions
- 1 tbsp. Kosher salt
- 1 handful finely chopped fresh parsley

For the batter

- 2 cups of water
- 3 cups all-purpose flour
- ¼ cup canola oil
- ½ tsp. Kosher salt
- 1 tsp. baking powder
- 1 egg

Directions:

1. Melt olive oil in a pan and then set it aside.
2. Cut the spinachinto pieces and lay them in a large bowl, then rinse and drain it in a small

spinner. Put the spinach back into that same bowl that you were using.

3. Add salt, pepper, scallions, onions, parsley, and garlic into the spinach bowl. Mix them well and add Feta cheese into the mixture, mixing all of that in, too.
4. Set these aside while you make the batter.
5. Measure the salt, baking powder, and 3 cups of flour into another smaller bowl. In the middle of the flour, form a crater and in it, put water, the unbeaten egg, and canola oil. Mix them all together until smooth.
6. Spread some of the oil into a roasting pan, and spread some of the batter on top of that.
7. You can take the eggs and beat them a bit. Then pour this into that spinach mixture you already did.
8. Evenly spoon and spread the spinach mixture into the baking pan.
9. Spoon the rest of the batter so that the spinach is covered. Then add the rest of the olive oil on top.
10. Turn on the oven and let it heat up to 350 degrees. Place the mixture into the oven and give it some time to bake. After 50 minutes, the dish should be done.
11. Allow it to cool before cutting it into squares and serving.

Easy Lunch Recipes to Get You in Shape

Tuna Patties

Cooking Time: 10 mins
Prep time: 15 mins

Ingredients:

- Lemon juice (2 Tbsp.)
- Parmesan cheese (3 Tbsp.)
- Pepper (1 pinch)
- Diced onion (3 Tbsp.)
- Canned tuna (3 cans)
- Italian seasoned breadcrumbs (10 Tbsp.)
- Olive oil (3 Tbsp.)
- Eggs (2)

Directions:

1. Whisk the lemon juice with the egg in a bowl. Then add in the bread crumbs and Parmesan cheese in order to make a nice paste.
2. Fold in the tuna and onion, and season with some pepper. Shape this mixture into tuna patties, about eight of them.
3. Heat the oil in a skillet. Fry the tuna patties until they turn golden brown. Serve.

Nutritional Information:

Calories 325
Fat: 15.5g
Carbs: 14g

Protein: 31.3g

Salmon Quinoa Burgers

Cooking Time: 15 mins
Prep time: 15 mins

Ingredients:

For burgers

- Old Bay (.5 tsp.)
- Dijon mustard (2 Tbsp.)
- Cooked quinoa (.75 c.)
- Pepper
- Salt
- Beaten egg (1)
- Chopped kale (1 c.)
- Diced shallots (.33 c.)
- Olive oil (1 tsp.)
- Wild salmon fillet (16 oz.)

Salad

- Olive oil (2.5 Tbsp.)
- Diced grapefruit (1)
- Baby arugula (10 c.)
- Pepper
- Salt
- Dijon mustard (1.25 tsp.)
- Minced shallots (2 Tbsp.0
- Champagne vinegar (2.5 Tbsp.)

Directions:

1. Bring out a bowl and whisk together the pepper, salt, Dijon, shallots, vinegar, and oil.
2. Cut off four pieces of the salmon and put it into the food processor to make it nice and fine. This helps to keep the burgers together.
3. Chop up the rest of the salmon and move them to a bowl. Heat up your skillet before adding the oil and cooking the kale and the shallots. Season and then heat until it becomes tender and wilted.
4. Move this to the bowl with the salmon and add the egg, Old Bay, Dijon, and quinoa. Combine them before forming them into 5 patties.
5. Prepare a grill pan or a skillet and then add in the salmon patties when it is hot. Cook these for five minutes before flipping. Continue to cook until done.
6. Toss the dressing you made with the grapefruit and arugula and then divide up on four plates. Top with a salmon burger and enjoy.

Nutritional Information:

Calories: 277
Fat: 13g
Carbs: 17g
Protein: 23g

Pasta with Smoked Salmon

Cooking Time: 15 mins
Prep Time: 15 mins

Ingredients:

- Chopped dill (1 Tbsp.)
- Salt (2.5 tsp.)
- Smoked salmon (8 oz.)
- Pepper (.25 tsp.)
- Capers (1 Tbsp.)
- Lemon zest (1 Tbsp.)
- Sliced scallions (3)
- Greek yogurt (1 c.)
- Olive oil (2 Tbsp.)
- Fettuccini (1 lb.)

Directions:

1. Cook up the noodles following the instructions on the package. Return the pasta back into the pot once it's drained. Add in the pepper, some salt, capers, lemon zest, scallions, yogurt, and olive oil and mix these well together.
2. Place this in a serving dish. Then arrange the salmon on top of it all.
3. Garnish the casserole with some olive oil and some dill before serving.

Nutritional Information:

Calories: 504
Fat: 13g
Carbs: 68g
Protein: 27g

Chicken and Rice Soup

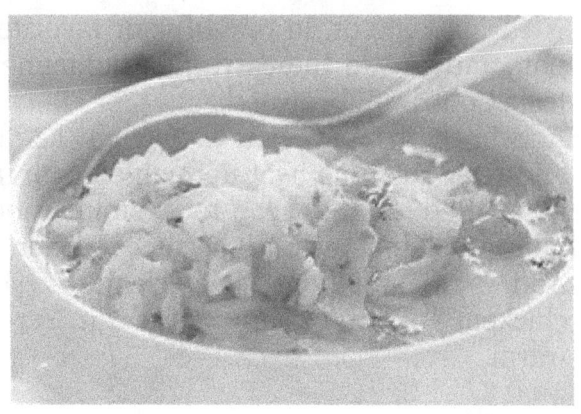

Cooking Time: 20 mins
Prep Time: 15 mins

Ingredients:

- Sliced scallions (2)
- Lemon juice (1)
- Cooked chicken (2 c.)
- Pepper
- Salt
- Fresh thyme (2 sprigs)
- Chicken broth (6 c.)
- Rice (.5 c.)
- Sliced carrots (2)
- Sliced garlic clove (1)
- Chopped fennel bulb (1)
- Sliced leek (2)
- Olive oil (.25 c.)

Directions:

1. Heat up some oil in one of your favorite soup pots and add in the carrot, garlic, fennel, and leek. Cook until browned.
2. Add in the pepper, salt, thyme, chicken broth, and rice. Turn the heat up high enough until it boils. Reduce the heat to a simmer once it boils. Cook the rice until becomes tender.
3. Add in the scallions, juice, lemon zest, and chicken. Take the thyme sprigs out. Serve this warm.

Nutritional Information:

Calories: 382
Fat: 15g
Carbs: 34g
Protein: 27g

Tuna and Egg Salad

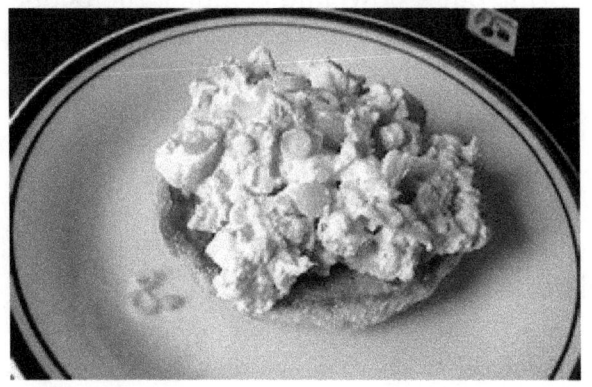

Prep Time: 20 mins

Ingredients:

- Pepper
- Salt
- Red wine vinegar (.25 c.)
- Capers (2 Tbsp.)
- Hard-boiled eggs (2)
- Nicoise olives (.5 c.)
- Minced garlic clove (1)
- Sliced red onion (.5)
- Sliced red bell pepper (1)
- Cubed tomatoes (4)
- Tuna (2 cans)
- Baby spinach (1 package)

Directions:

1. Bring out a bowl and combine the pepper, salt, vinegar, olive oil, capers, eggs, olives, garlic, onion, bell pepper, tomatoes, tuna, and spinach. Toss to mix well.
2. Let this set for about ten minutes to marinate the flavors together.
3. Place into a serving bowl and then serve.

Nutritional Information:

Calories: 340
Fat: 23g
Carbs: 11g
Protein: 24g

Fennel and Crab Salad

Prep Time: 15 mins

Ingredients:

- Red pepper flakes (.25 tsp.)
- Chopped parsley (2 Tbs.)
- Juice and zest from a lemon
- Dijon mustard (1 tsp.)
- Minced shallot (1)
- Olive oil (.33 c.)
- Pepper
- Salt
- Crabmeat (1 lb.)
- Pink grapefruit, cubed (1)
- Sliced fennel bulb (1)
- Chopped Romaine lettuce (1 head)

Directions:

1. In a platter, place the lettuce properly and top it the grapefruit, crab meat, and fennel. Sprinkle on the pepper and the salt.
2. Whisk the salt, red pepper flakes, lemon juice, parsley, and zest, mustard, shallot, and olive oil in a small bowl.
3. Sprinkle the mixture over the salad and then serve.

Nutritional Information:

Calories: 294
Fat: 18g
Carbs: 27g
Protein: 10g

Zucchini Panini

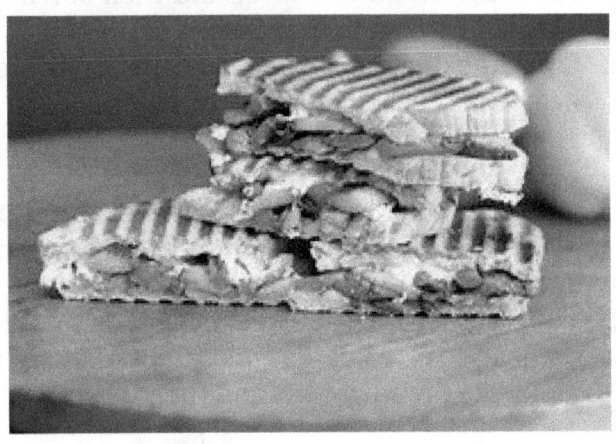

Cooking Time: 10 mins
Prep Time: 15 mins

Ingredients:

- Sliced manchego cheese (4 oz.)
- Baby spinach (2 c.)
- Red pepper flakes (.25 tsp.)
- Salt
- Sliced mushrooms (8)
- Sliced zucchini (2)
- Olive oil (.25 c.)
- Dijon mustard (2 tsp.)
- Italian bread (8 slices)

Directions:

1. Place the bread in a layer and then spread four of them with some mustard.
2. Over the high heat temperature of the oven, heat up the skillet. Add in the olive oil, red pepper flakes, salt, mushrooms, and zucchini. Let these cook until they are tender.
3. Divide up the vegetables between four bread pieces and then top with the slices of the cheese and spinach.
4. Top these with the other slices of bread and then add to a hot Panini or a skillet. Grill to make the bread golden and then serve.

Nutritional Information:

Calories: 313
Fat: 24g
Carbs: 16g
Protein: 12g

Greek Village Salad

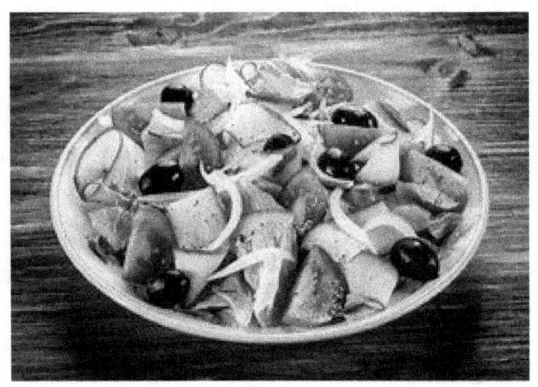

Prep Time: 15 mins

Ingredients:

- Dried oregano (1 tsp.)
- Feta cheese (4 oz.)
- Kalamata olives (.5 c.)
- Red wine vinegar (2 Tbsp.)
- Pepper (.25 tsp.)
- Salt (1 tsp.)
- Sliced red onion (.5)
- Olive oil (.25 c.)
- Sliced tomatoes (3)
- Sliced cucumbers (2)

Directions:

1. Bring out a platter and arrange the cucumbers as the first layer. Top the cucumbers with the other vegetables.
2. Sprinkle on the pepper and salt and drizzle the red wine vinegar and olive oil on top of everything.
3. Scatter out the olives and put the feta in the middle before serving.

Nutritional Information:

Calories: 263
Fat: 20g
Carbs: 15g
Protein: 7g

Chicken Corn Salad

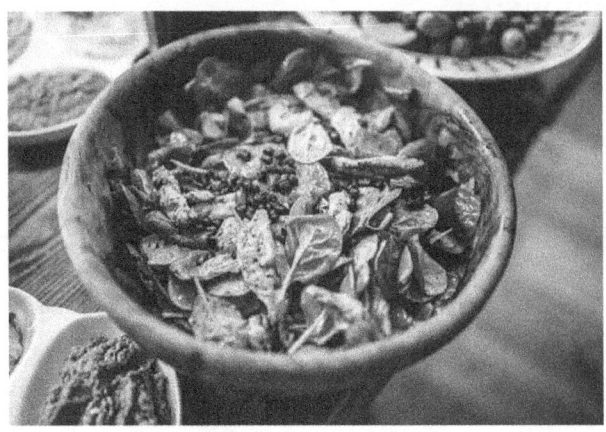

Cooking Time: 25 mins
Prep Time: 10 mins

Ingredients:

- Corn kernels (2 ears)
- Chopped onion (.5 c.)
- Chicken breasts (2)
- Lemon juice (.25 c. and 1 Tbsp.)
- Cilantro leaves (2 Tbsp.)
- Flour (.33 c.)
- Diced yellow tomato (1)
- Pepper
- Dijon mustard (1 Tbsp.)
- Salt
- Diced summer squash (1)
- Olive oil (3 Tbsp.)
- Minced jalapeno chili (1)

Directions:

1. Mix together 0.25 cup of lemon juice with the mustard. Slice up each chicken breast in half to get two fillets and add to the mustard mixture. Make sure that both sides get coated.
2. Heat up your oil to make it hot before adding in the onion. Then add in the squash, chili, and corn. Cook them for about 15 minutes until they get soft.
3. Take the pan from the heat and fold in the rest of the lemon juice with the tomatoes.
4. Take the chicken out of the marinade and dust with the flour. Season it with the pepper and salt as well.
5. Sear the chicken in the heated oil in a grill pan, turning just once.
6. When the chicken is done, arrange on a platter and then add cooking oil to your salad before spooning the mixture all over the chicken and the rest of the ingredients.

Nutritional Information:

Calories: 449
Fat: 24g
Carbs: 25g
Protein: 34g

Chicken Fried Rice

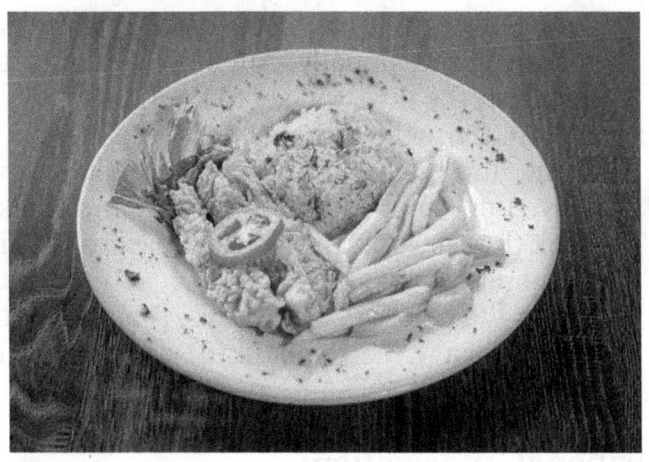

Cooking Time: 15 mins
Prep Time: 10 mins

Ingredients:

- Soy sauce (3 Tbsp.)
- Frozen green peas (.5 c.)
- Brown rice, cooked (2 c.)
- Diced carrots (.5 c.)
- Chicken breast, cubed (12 oz.)
- Minced garlic cloves (2)
- Chopped scallion (.5 c.)
- Egg white (4)
- Cooking spray

Directions:

1. Use the cooking spray to coat your skillet before heating it up. Cook the egg whites and stir them occasionally. After five minutes, take this from the heat and set to the side.
2. Recoat the skillet some more and heat it up again. Add the garlic and scallions and let these warm up. Then, add in the carrots and chicken. Cook these so that the chicken reaches the right temperature.
3. Stir in the reserved egg whites, peas, soy sauce, and brown rice. Cook until warm and then serve.

Nutritional Information:

Calories: 179
Fat: 2g
Carbs: 21g
Protein: 18g

Turkey Tacos

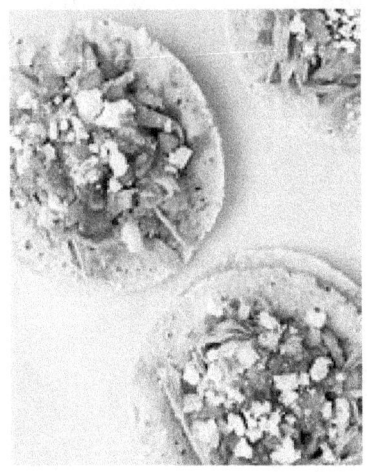

Prep Time: 14 mins
Cooking Time: 1 min

Ingredients:

- Cranberry pear sauce (8 Tbsp.)
- Cooked turkey, shredded (12 oz.)
- Whole wheat tortillas (8)
- Lemon juice (2 tsp.)
- Sliced Brussels sprouts (8)
- Pepper
- Salt
- Olive oil (.5 Tbsp.)

Directions:

1. Bring out a bowl and whisk your salt, oil, pepper, and lemon juice together. Add in the onion and the Brussels sprouts and toss to coat.
2. If you would like to heat up the tortillas, then do so. Then top each one with some turkey, some of the slaw, and the cranberry sauce.

Nutritional Information:

Calories: 235
Fat: 5g
Carbs: 30g
Protein: 21.5g

Asparagus and Pork

Cooking Time: 30 mins
Prep Time: 5 mins

Ingredients:

- Apple cider vinegar (2 Tbsp.)
- Sliced shallot (3)
- Trimmed asparagus (1 lb.)
- Salt
- Whole-grain mustard (1 Tbsp.)
- Pork tenderloin (1.25 lbs.)
- Olive oil (.33 c. and 2 Tbsp.)
- Pepper

Directions:

1. Turn on the oven and let it heat up to 400 degrees. Make sure that the skillet is nice and warm and then add in the oil. Season all the pieces of pork with some pepper and salt. Cook it and make sure that it is browned.
2. Move the skillet into your oven and let the pork roast until it is cooked through. After 15 minutes, take the pork out of the oven and then let it rest before slicing.
3. Bring out a sheet that you can bake with and toss the shallots and asparagus with some oil before you season them.
4. Place the vegetables evenly onto your sheet so that they cook the right way. After 15 minutes, take them out and let them cool down.

5. Whisk together the rest of the oil in a bowl with a bit of vinegar and mustard to make a dressing. Serve this over the vegetables and pork and enjoy.

Nutritional Information:

Calories: 476
Fat: 32g
Carbs: 8g
Protein: 39g

Pork Chops

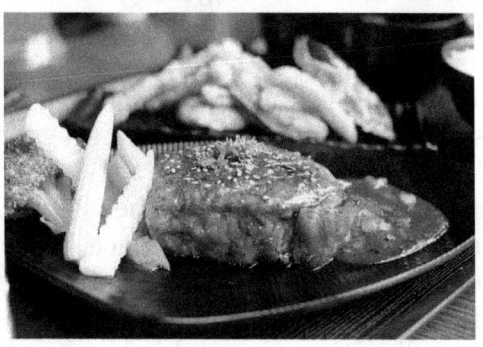

Cooking Times: 25 mins
Prep Time: 10 mins

Ingredients:

- Chicken seasoning (.75 tsp.)
- Pork chops, sliced (16 oz.)
- Lemon rind (1 tsp.)
- Juice from a lemon
- Feta cheese (.25 c.)
- Sliced Kalamata olives (.25 c.)
- Sliced garlic cloves (3)
- Oregano (.25 tsp.)
- Pepper
- Olive oil (1 Tbsp.)
- Tomatoes (1 c.)
- Trimmed yellow squash (6 oz.)
- Trimmed zucchini (6 oz.)

Directions:

1. Turn on the oven to 450 degrees and let it heat up. Season the pork chops with the chicken seasoning.
2. Slice up the yellow squash and zucchini. Then toss the tomatoes with some oregano, pepper, salt, and olive oil.
3. Place these tomatoes, cut the side up, and then spray with cooking oil. Place these into the oven and roast it. After ten minutes, add the garlic and roast for an additional 5 minutes.
4. Move all of these into a big bowl and set to the side. Reduce the heat to 200 degrees.
5. Heat up a skillet and then place the zucchini inside with some oil and a little salt. Cook until tender. Add this to the tomatoes and place in a warm oven.
6. Working in a few batches, cook up half your pork chops for a few minutes on both sides.
7. Make sure that the vegetables are taken out when they are done and toss in the lemon rind and juice and the olives. Serve these over the pork chops and top with the Feta cheese to enjoy.

Nutritional Information:

Calories: 230
Fat: 9g
Carbs: 9g
Protein: 28g

Chicken Tostados

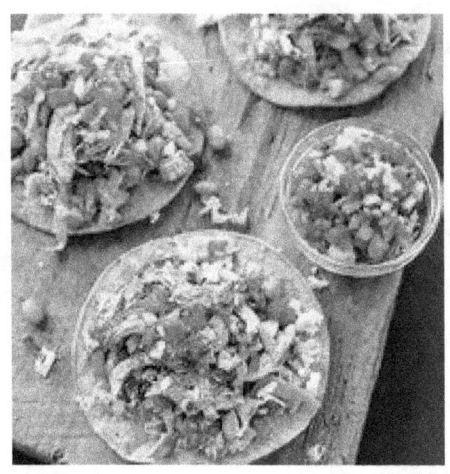

Cooking Time: 45 mins
Prep time: 10 mins

Ingredients:

- Minced red onion (.5)
- Chopped green chilies (4.5 oz.)
- Red wine vinegar (1 Tbsp.)
- Chicken thighs (2 lbs.)
- Sour cream (.25 c.)
- Shredded Monterey Jack cheese (1 c.)
- Chopped scallions (8)
- Refried beans (1 c.)
- Whole wheat tortillas (8)
- Barbecue sauce (1 c.)
- Diced tomatoes (2)
- Salt
- Olive oil (2 Tbsp.)
- Minced garlic clove (1)

- Chopped cilantro (.25 c.)

Directions:

1. Combine together the chilies, barbecue sauce, and chicken in a pan and let them boil. When it boils, lower the heat. For the next twenty-five minutes, simmer the chicken until it is done.
2. During this time, bring out a bowl and combine the salt, oil, vinegar, garlic, cilantro, onion, and tomatoes. Set to the side.
3. Turn on the oven and let it heat up to 425 degrees. Prepare a baking sheet and pour the tortilla chips on top of it all.
4. Spread evenly the chicken and the beans on top of your tortillas .Place them in the oven.
5. After fifteen minutes, everything should be done, so take it out of the oven. Top with the tomato mixture, sour cream, and more cilantro and then serve.

Nutritional Information:

Calories: 307
Fat: 5g
Carbs: 15g
Protein: 32g

Caprese Wrap

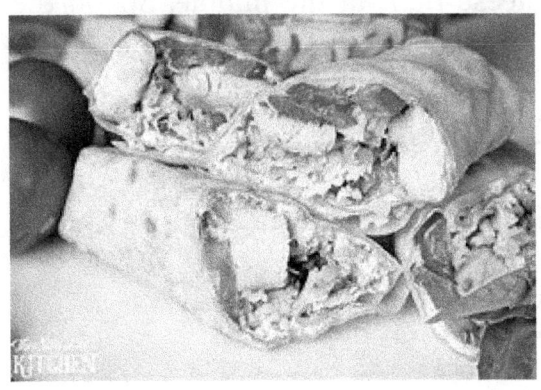

Cooking Time: 0 min
Prep Time: 20 mins

Ingredients:

- Mozzarella cheese (6 oz.)
- Sandwich wraps (4)
- Red wine vinegar (1 Tbsp.)
- Chopped basil (.25 c.)
- Red pepper flakes (.25 tsp.)
- Salt (1 tsp.)
- Olive oil (.25 c.)
- Sliced cherry tomatoes (.5 pint)

Directions:

1. Bring out a bowl and mix together the basil, red pepper flakes, salt, red wine vinegar, olive oil, and tomatoes.

2. Place the wraps on a work surface and place the cheese right in the middle. Spoon the tomato mixture on top and fold the wrap so that it encloses the filling.
3. Place the seam side down and let it rest a bit to marinate before serving.

Nutritional Information:

Calories: 291
Fat: 21g
Carbs: 14g
Protein: 14g

Aram Sandwich

Prep Time: 30 mins
Cooking Time: 0 min

Ingredients:

- Chopped scallions (.5 c.)
- Green olives (.25 c.)
- Chopped red peppers, roasted (.5 c.)
- Spinach (1 c.)
- Hummus (1 c.)
- Lavash (2 pieces)
- Sliced cucumbers (1 c.)

Directions:

1. Place your lavash on the work surface and spread out the hummus on each one. Arrange the spinach on the lower part of each bread piece.
2. Top with the cucumbers, roasted peppers, green olives, and scallions. Roll this up from the bottom until it ends up like a jelly roll.
3. Put it inside a plastic wrap and place into the fridge until you are ready to serve. Slice it up before serving.

Nutritional Information:

Calories: 237
Fat: 10g
Carbs: 32g
Protein: 9g

Grilled Veggie Wrap

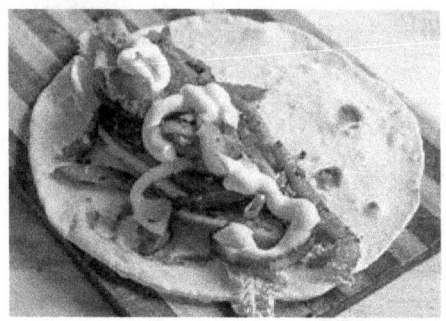

Prep Time: 20 mins

Ingredients:

- Pepper
- Salt
- Lemon juice (3 tsp.)
- Parsley (.25 c.)
- Sliced red onion (1)
- Baby spinach (1 c.)
- Tapenade (.25 c.)
- Olive oil (.25 c.)
- Sandwich wraps (4)
- Sliced red bell pepper (1)
- Sliced zucchini (3)

Directions:

1. Heat up your grill. Brush the onion, bell pepper, and zucchini with some oil before grilling a few minutes on both sides. Move the

vegetables from the grill and cover with foil so that they can steam for the next five minutes.
2. Arrange your wraps on a work surface. Place the vegetables in the middle of these wraps before topping with the pepper, salt, lemon juice, parsley, spinach, and tapenade.
3. Fold the wrap on the filling and place the seam side down. Serve when ready.

Nutritional Information:

Calories: 240
Fat: 17g
Carbs: 21g
Protein: 4g

Tomato and Feta Ciabatta

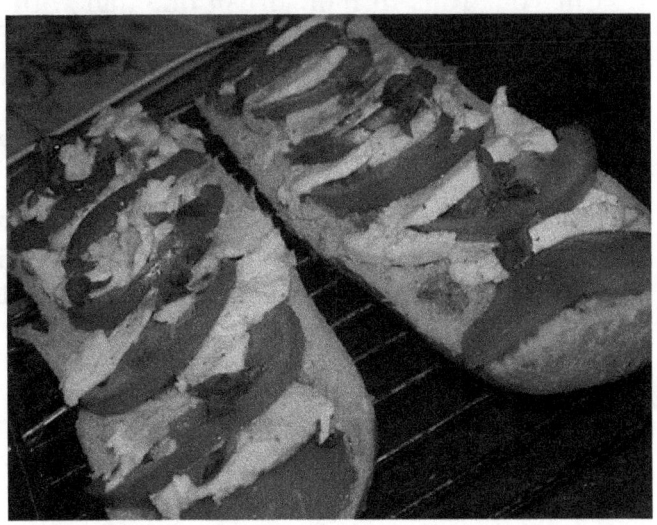

Prep Time: 15 mins

Ingredients:

- Pepper
- Oregano (1 tsp.)
- Salt
- Crumbled feta cheese (4 oz.)
- Red wine vinegar (2 Tbsp.)
- English cucumber (16 slices)
- Sliced tomatoes (3)
- Tapenade (.25 c.)
- Olive oil (.5 c.)
- Ciabatta (4)

Directions:
1. Cut your rolls in half. Brush one half with the vinegar and olive oil. On the second half of each roll, spread some of the tapenade on it.
2. Place a few slices of tomato over the tapenade and then top with some cucumbers and feta cheese on top.
3. Sprinkle each of the sandwiches with the pepper, oregano, and salt. Top with the other half of the ciabatta roll and let them marinate a few minutes before serving.

Nutritional Information:

Calories: 450
Fat: 36g
Carbs: 24g
Protein: 9g

Tuscan Tuna Pita

Cooking Time: 0 mins
Prep Time: 20 mins

Ingredients:

- Pepper
- Salt
- Pepperoncini (.25 c.)
- Pesto (.25 c.)
- Red onion, chopped (.5 c.)
- Roasted red peppers (.25 c.)
- White beans, cooked (1 c.)
- Tuna (2 cans)
- Red wine vinegar (1 Tbsp.)
- Shredded romaine lettuce (1 c.)
- Whole wheat pita bread (4)

Directions:

1. Cut each of your pita bread in half through the middle. Tuck the romaine into the bottom of each pita to help keep them over when it's time to stuff them up.
2. Bring out a bowl and combine the red onion, roasted peppers, white beans, tuna, pesto, pepperoncini, pepper, salt, and vinegar.
3. Stuff this mixture into the pitas and then serve.

Nutritional Information:

Calories: 456
Fat: 14g

Carbs: 54g
Protein: 33g

Lamb Mint Sliders

Cooking Time: 15 mins
Prep Time: 15 mins

Ingredients:

- Roma tomatoes (8 slices)
- Chopped mint (2 Tbsp.)
- Mayo (.5 c.)
- Pepper
- Red onion (8 slices)
- Salt
- Balsamic vinegar (1 Tbsp>)
- Minced garlic clove (1)
- Ground lamb (2 lbs.)
- Dinner rolls (8)

Directions:

1. Grab each roll and cut it in half. Then bring out a bowl and combine the pepper, salt, vinegar, garlic, and lamb together. After you have made sure that the ingredients are mixed well, use your hands to make eight patties out of the mixture.
2. Heat up a frying pan and add in a bit of oil. Add your lamb patties onto the grill and cook each side for about four minutes.
3. Take the lamb patties out of the heat and let them rest while you work on the mint mayo.
4. Combine together your mayo and mint to make the dressing. Spread this dressing on both

pieces of bread and then make sure the lamb patty is on the bottom.
5. Top with a slice of red onion and tomato before serving.

Nutritional Information:

Calories: 682
Fat: 29g
Carbs: 34g
Protein: 69g

Mushroom Pesto Pizza

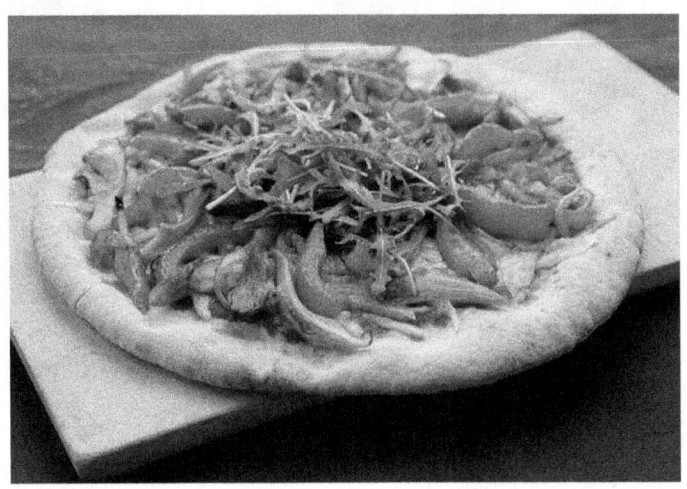

Cooking Time: 15 mins
Prep Time: 15 mins

Ingredients:

- Shredded cheese (.5 c.)
- Pesto (.5 c.)
- Whole wheat pita bread (4)
- Red pepper flakes (.25 tsp.)
- Salt
- Sliced mushrooms (12)
- Olive oil (.25 c.)

Directions:

1. Turn on the oven and let it heat up to 375 degrees. Warm up a skillet and then add in the

red pepper flakes, salt, mushrooms, and olive oil.
2. Let these ingredients cook until they are nice and tender.
3. Make sure the pita bread is on your baking sheet before topping it with a good layer of pesto. Add on the cheese and the mushrooms and then put your sheet inside the oven to bake.
4. After 15 minutes, the pizza should be browned and you can serve it right away.

Nutritional Information:

Calories: 474
Fat: 31g
Carbs: 40g
Protein: 16g

Dinner Meals for the Whole Family

Easy Tuna Salad

Cooking Time: 0 min
Prep Time: 15 mins

Ingredients:

- Pepper
- Salt
- Celery seed (.5 tsp.)
- Honey mustard (2 tsp.)
- Dill pickle relish (1.5 Tbsp.)
- Mayo (.75 c.)
- Chopped celery stalk (1)
- Sweet onion, chopped (.5 c.)
- Chopped hard-boiled eggs (5)
- Canned tuna (4 cans)

Directions:

1. Bring out a big bowl and combine the celery, onion, eggs, and tuna together.
2. In another bowl, stir together the pepper, salt, celery seed, honey mustard, relish, and mayo.
3. Pour the ingredients in this second bowl over the ones in the first bowl. Stir around to coat and serve.

Nutritional Information:

Calories: 186
Fat: 13.6g
Carbs: 2g
Protein: 13.6g

Grilled Salmon Kebabs

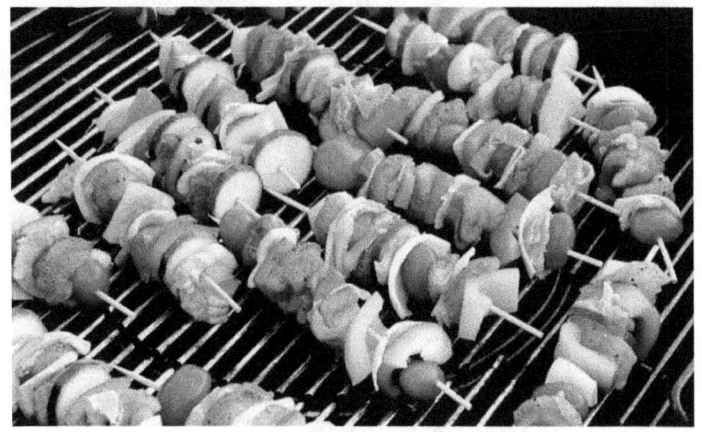

Cooking Time: 10 mins
Prep Time: 10 mins

Ingredients:

- Salt
- Sesame seeds (2 tsp.)
- Cooking spray
- Sliced lemons (2)
- Sliced salmon fillets (1.5 lbs.)
- Red pepper flakes (.25 tsp.)
- Chopped oregano (2 Tbsp.)
- Cumin (1 tsp.)

Directions:

1. Heat up the grill and add some cooking spray onto it. While that heats up, mix together the red pepper flakes, cumin, sesame seeds, and oregano in a bowl.
2. Starting and then ending with the salmon, thread alternately the salmon and the lemon slices onto eight of the skewers to make eight kebabs.
3. Make sure to coat the salmon with some oil before seasoning.
4. Grill the fish for 10minutes. Serve.

Nutritional Information:

Calories: 267
Fat: 11g
Carbs: 7g
Protein: 35g

Cilantro Tilapia

Cooking Time: 12 mins
Prep Time: 5 mins

Ingredients:

- Cilantro (1 bunch)
- Pepper
- Cajun seasoning (2 Tbsp.)
- Garlic salt (2 Tbsp.)
- Tilapia fillets (4)
- Olive oil (3 Tbsp.)

Directions:

1. Turn on the oven and allow it to heat up to 375 degrees. Bring out a baking dish and coat it with some olive oil. Add the tilapia pieces into this prepared pan.
2. Sprinkle some pepper, Cajun seasoning, and garlic salt on top of your tilapia pieces and then press in some of the cilantro sprigs onto each piece.
3. Place the tilapia into the oven. After 12 minutes, the tilapia is done and you can enjoy!

Nutritional Information:

Calories: 200
Fat: 12.1g

Carbs: .3g
Protein: 23g

Shrimp Skewers

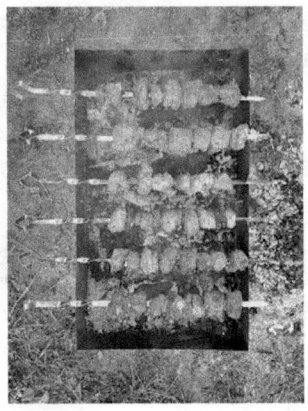

Cooking Time: 5 mins
Prep Time: 15 mins

Ingredients:

- Skewers
- Chopped cilantro (.25 c.)
- Paprika (.25 tsp.)
- Pepper
- Salt
- Lime juice (.25 c.)
- Olive oil (2 Tbsp.)
- Sliced garlic cloves (3)
- Shrimp (1 lb.)

Directions:

1. Bring out a bowl and make your marinade by whisking together the paprika, pepper, salt, garlic, lime juice, and olive oil.
2. Thread your shrimp onto the skewers. Place about five or six shrimps on each skewer. Add to a plate before pouring the marinade on top of the shrimp.
3. You can grill these by adding the skewers to a preheated grill and cooking so that both sides get grilled well. Add the extra marinade as a baster as you go.

Nutritional Information:

Calories: 108
Fat: 5g
Carbs: 1g
Protein: 15g

Chicken with Mushrooms

Cooking Time: 30 mins
Prep Time: 10 mins

Ingredients:

- Olive oil (3 Tbsp.)
- Chopped thyme leaves (2 Tbsp.)
- Milk (.75 c.)
- Flour (2 Tbsp.)
- Diced onion (.5 c.)
- Baby Bell mushrooms (2 c.)
- Chicken breasts (4)
- Pepper
- Salt
- Minced garlic cloves (1)

Directions:

1. Even up the thickness of the chicken by pounding the bottom of the glass into it. Salt and pepper the chicken breast.
2. Bring out a pan and make sure that it is coated well with the olive oil. Place the chicken in the pan and cook until golden. Turn the chicken over and reduce the heat on the stove.
3. Place the lid tightly onto the pan and let this cook. Let the pan cool for 10 minutes with the lid on once cooked.
4. Check the chicken when this is done to make sure it reaches 165 degrees. When it reaches that temperature, take it out of the pan to cool down.

5. Cook the onion and the mushrooms next. When they are done, thicken them using some flour.
6. Heat the garlic on the pan as well. Then add in the pepper, salt, thyme, and milk. Whisk the mixture. Repeat until the sauce is thick.
7. Add the chicken to a serving plate and pour the sauce on top before serving.

Nutritional Information:

Calories: 315
Fat: 16g
Carbs: 8g
Protein: 35g

Tomato and Chicken Salad

Cooking Time: 20 mins
Prep Time: 20 mins

Ingredients:

- Olive oil (.25 c.)
- Pitted Kalamata olives (12)
- Tomatoes, sliced (1 lb.)
- Red onion, sliced (1)
- Pepper
- Salt
- Chicken breast (.5 lbs.)
- Romaine Lettuce (1 heart)
- Mint leaves (4 Tbsp.)
- Crumbled feta cheese (2 oz.)
- Red wine vinegar (1 Tbsp.)
- Lemon juice (1 Tbsp.)

Directions:

1. Turn on the oven and heat it up so that it can reach 400 degrees. Toss the chicken into a bowl with some oil, salt, and pepper.
2. Turn on a grill pan and then sear the chicken on it for a few minutes on each side. Move to a baking pan and place into the oven.
3. Test the chicken after 15 minutes to see if it is at 165 degrees. When the chicken is done, take it off the heat and give it time to cool down.
4. Use some water on a bowl to soak the onion. After five minutes drain out the water.

5. When the chicken is cool enough, tear it up a bit and then make sure it goes into the same bowl again. Add in the olives, tomatoes, and onion. Season with pepper and salt and toss in the rest of the vinegar, olive oil, and lemon juice. Add the feta and mint and toss some more.
6. Line a platter or a bowl with some lettuce and top with the tomato salad and chicken.

Nutritional Information:

Calories: 278
Fat: 19g
Carbs: 10g
Protein: 17g

Lemony Chicken

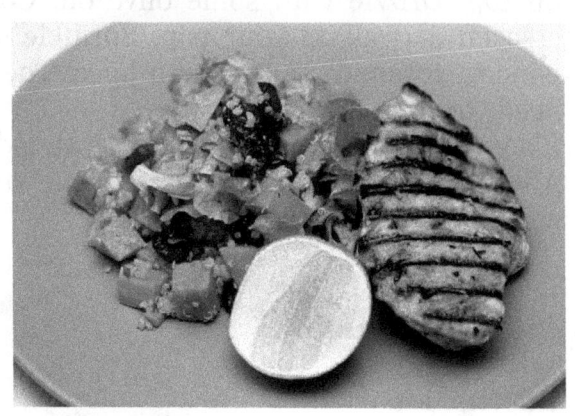

Cooking Time: 35 mins
Prep Time: 10 mins

Ingredients:

- Salt
- Chopped rosemary (2 tsp.)
- Chicken breast (1 lb.)
- Quartered lemon (1)
- Lemon juice (2 tsp.)
- Pepper
- Chicken broth (.25 c.)
- Olive oil (1 tsp.)
- Chopped parsley (2 tsp.)

Directions:

1. Turn on the oven and heat up to 400 degrees. While that warms up, use the pepper and salt to season the chicken.

2. Bring out a roasting pan and place the chicken on top. Drizzle with some olive oil. Coat the chicken as well as your pan. Sprinkle on the parsley, rosemary, and lemon juice. The broth needs to go in next.
3. Place the pan in the oven when it's already hot. After 30 minutes, the chicken is done and you can serve with a bit of lemon

Nutritional Information:

Calories: 146
Fat: 4g
Carbs: 1g
Protein: 25g

Chicken Rollatini

Cooking Time: 25 mins
Prep Time: 10 mins

Ingredients:

- Romano cheese (.25 c.)
- Seasoned breadcrumbs (.5 c.)
- Sliced red onion (.25 c.)
- Olive oil (1 Tbsp.)
- Shredded mozzarella (.5 c.)
- Dried tomato bruschetta (.5 c.)
- Lemon juice (1)
- Sliced chicken cutlets (8)

Directions:

1. Bring out a bowl and combine the cheese with the breadcrumbs. Combine the oil, pepper, and the lemon juice together well.
2. Turn on the oven and let it heat up to 450 degrees.
3. Place each of the cutlets on a cutting board and add some red onion, spinach leaves, mozzarella cheese, and bruschetta in the middle. Roll and place the seam side down on a work surface.
4. Repeat this with all the chicken. Dip the pieces into the lemon-oil mixture before adding into the mixture with the breadcrumbs. Add to a cooking sheet when they are coated.

5. Place these into the oven and let them bake. After 25 minutes, take the chicken out and serve.

Nutritional Information:

Calories: 267
Fat: 14g
Carbs: 10g
Protein: 25g

Greek Turkey Burgers

Cooking Time: 10 mins
Prep Time: 20 mins

Ingredients:

- Feta cheese (.25 c.)
- Pepper
- Salt
- Oregano (1 Tbsp.)
- Red onion, grated (2 Tbsp.)
- Whole wheat breadcrumbs (.25 c.)
- Ground turkey (1 lb.)
- Grated zucchini (5 oz.)

Salad Ingredients

- Crumbled feta (1 Tbsp.)
- Salt
- Roasted peppers (.25 c.)
- Olive oil (1 tsp.)
- Kalamata olives (.33 c.)
- Chopped red onion (2 Tbsp.)
- Oregano (1 tsp.)
- Quartered grape tomatoes (.75 c.)
- Diced cucumber (1)
- Red wine vinegar (2 tsp.)

Directions:

1. Squeeze out the moisture from the zucchini. Then combine it together with the pepper, salt, oregano, onion, garlic, breadcrumbs, and ground turkey.
2. Mix those ingredients well and then add in some feta cheese. Divide this into five patties and store in the fridge.
3. In another bowl, combine the rest of the feta with the salt, vinegar, red onion, tomato, and cucumber.
4. Heat up a skillet on the stove and when it is hot, add on some oil. Place the burgers in the pan and reduce the heat a bit.
5. Cook the burgers on one side until brown and then flip. Flip a few times to prevent burning while also ensuring that they cook evenly.

Nutritional Information:

Calories: 221
Fat: 11g
Carbs: 10g
Protein: 20g

Mussels with Garlic and Wine

Cooking Time: 20 mins
Prep Time: 10 mins

Ingredients:

- Chopped parsley (1 Tbsp.)
- Salt
- White wine (2 c.)
- Mussels (4 lbs.)
- Minced garlic cloves (2)
- Olive oil (3 Tbsp.)

Directions:

1. Add a heavy pot to the stove. Add in the seasonings and the oil and let them cook for a few minutes.
2. When those are warm, toss in the rest of the ingredients. Let the boil inside the pot. When the mussels boil, reduce the heat to a simmer.
3. If there are any mussels that aren't opened at this time, discard them. Serve this with the juices and enjoy.

Nutritional Information:

Calories: 581
Fat: 21g
Carbs: 21g
Protein: 54g

Shrimp Scampi

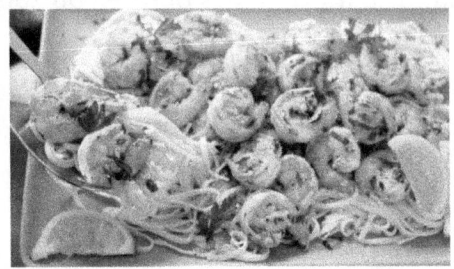

Cooking Time: 10 mins
Prep Time: 15 mins

Ingredients:

- Lemon zest (1 Tbsp.)
- Chopped parsley (1 Tbsp.)
- Salt
- Dry vermouth (.25 c.)
- Minced garlic clove (1)
- Lemon juice (2 Tbsp.)
- Jump shrimp (1.5 lbs.)
- Olive oil (2 Tbsp.)
- Butter (2 Tbsp.)

Directions:

1. Heat up some oil in a skillet before adding the butter. When your butter has melted, add in the garlic and shrimp and fry for a minute.
2. Then put in the salt and the vermouth and simmer a bit longer until you see the shrimp is cooked through.

3. Take the skillet off the heat. Then add in the remaining ingredients before you serve.

Nutritional Information:

Calories: 252
Fat: 13g
Carbs: 1g
Protein: 31g

Chicken Cacciatore

Cooking Time: 4 hours
Prep Time: 10 mins

Ingredients:

- Dried oregano (2 tsp.)
- Chicken broth (1 c.)
- Chopped red bell pepper (1)
- Crushed tomatoes (1 can)
- Red wine (.5 c.)
- Sliced garlic cloves (3)
- Chopped onion (1)
- Olive oil (2 Tbsp.)
- Pepper
- Capers (1 Tbsp.)
- Salt
- Chicken thighs (8)

Directions:

1. Place the chicken in the bottom of the slow cooker and sprinkle with the pepper and salt.
2. In a bowl, combine together the oregano, capers, chicken broth, tomatoes, red wine, garlic, bell pepper, onion, and olive oil. Pour this mixture on top of your chicken.
3. Place the lid on top. Cook them for four hours over high setting.

Nutritional Information:

Calories: 572
Fat: 32g
Carbs: 23g
Protein: 41g

Stuffed Chicken Breasts

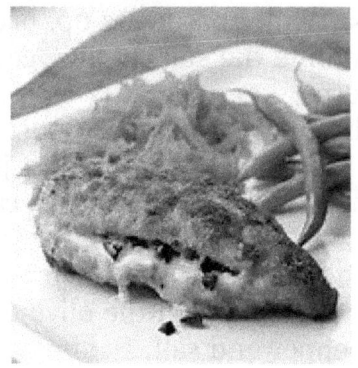

Cooking Time: 45 mins
Prep Time: 30 mins

Ingredients:

- Lemon (.5)
- White wine (1 c.)
- Pepper
- Olive oil (2 Tbsp>0
- Chicken breasts (4)
- Salt
- Thyme, chopped (.5 tsp.)
- Chopped garlic clove (1)
- Sun-dried tomatoes (2 Tbsp>)
- Ricotta cheese (4 oz.)

Directions:

1. Heat up the oven so that it can reach 375 degrees. While that heats up, bring out a bowl and combine the salt, thyme, garlic, tomatoes, and ricotta.
2. Place the chicken on a work surface. Slide your fingers into the skin and pull it just a bit away from the chicken breast, taking care to not tear it.
3. Add into the baking dish the breast stuffed with fillings. Sprinkle with the olive oil and the rest of the pepper and salt. Fill up the pan with the wine.
4. Put the whole dish into the oven and let it bake. After 45 minutes, you can remove your chicken breast from your oven. Sprinkle some of the juice from the lemon and enjoy.

Nutritional Information:

Calories: 359
Fat: 17g
Carbs: 4g
Protein: 37g

Pork Loin Gremolata

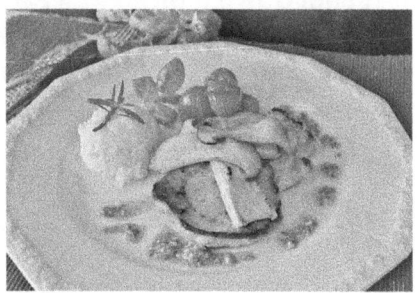

Cooking Time: 40 mins
Prep Time: 15 mins

Ingredients:

- Gremolata (1 recipe)
- Nutmeg (.25 tsp.)
- Pepper
- Salt
- Olive oil (2 Tbsp.)
- Pork loin roast (3 lbs.)
- Water (1 c.)

Directions:

1. Turn on the oven and let it heat up to 400 degrees. Take out a roasting pan and add a cup of water inside.
2. Rub your roast with some olive oil. It should be seasoned with the pepper, salt, and nutmeg. Place it into the oven.

3. After 40 minutes, take the roast out of the oven and let it cool down a bit.
4. When ready to serve, slice up the pork roast and spoon some Gremolata on the top before eating.

Nutritional Information:

Calories: 576
Fat: 22g
Carbs: 2g
Protein: 90g

Lamb Meatballs

Cooking Time: 15 mins
Prep Time: 15 mins

Ingredients:

- Salt (1 tsp.)
- Pepper
- Red pepper flakes (.25 tsp.)
- Cumin (.5 tsp.)
- Egg (1)
- Rice flour (3 Tbsp.)
- Dried oregano (1 tsp.)
- Minced garlic cloves (2)
- Sliced scallions (3)
- Ground lamb (1 lb.)

Directions:

1. Turn on the oven and let it heat up to 400 degrees. Bring out a bowl and place the red pepper flakes, cumin, salt, oregano, egg, rice flour, garlic, scallions, and lamb together inside.
2. Prepare a baking sheet. Use your hands or a small ice cream scoop to scoop the meatballs. Put the meatballs on the baking sheet. Place the meatballs into the oven.
3. After 15 minutes, the meatballs should be cooked through and firm. Allow them some

time to cool before arranging on a platter and serving.

Nutritional Information:

Calories: 262
Fat: 10g
Carbs: 8g
Protein: 34g

Pomegranate Lamb Shanks

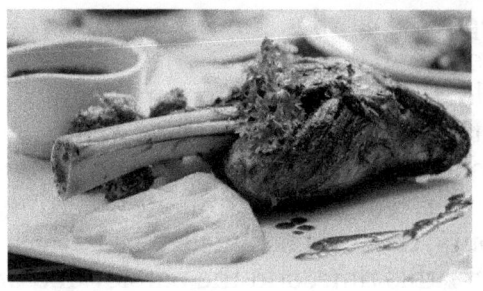

Cooking Time: 6 hours
Prep Time: 15 mins

Ingredients:

- Chopped parsley (.25 c.)
- Orange zest (1 Tbsp.)
- Honey (.25 c.)
- Pomegranate juice (1 c.)
- Minced garlic cloves (2)
- Chopped carrots (2)
- Olive oil (2 Tbsp.)
- Chopped onion (1)
- Pepper
- Paprika (1 tsp.)
- Salt (2 tsp.)
- Lamb shanks (4)

Directions:

1. Take the lamb shanks and season with the pepper, paprika, and salt. Add to the slow cooker.
2. Add the honey, pomegranate juice, olive oil, garlic, carrots, and onion as well.
3. Make sure that the lid is secure on the slow cooker. Turn this into its low setting. After six hours, the meal is done.
4. After this time, add the parsley and orange zest and then serve warm.

Nutritional Information:

Calories: 883
Fat: 52g
Carbs: 34g
Protein: 64g

Polenta Lasagna

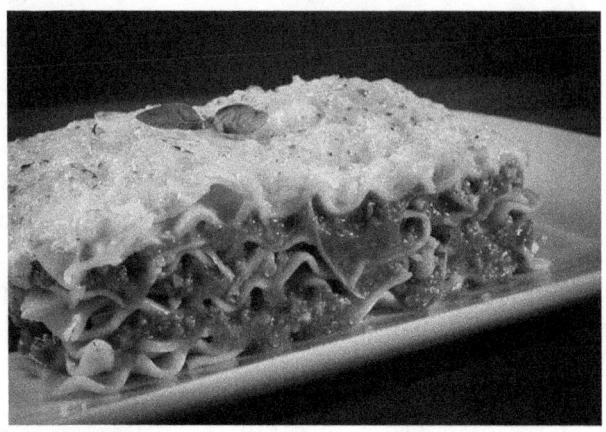

Cooking Time: 30 mins
Prep Time: 30 mins

Ingredients:

- Chopped rosemary (2 Tbsp.)
- Parmesan cheese (1 c.)
- Sliced mozzarella cheese (8 oz.)
- Sliced garlic cloves (2)
- Sliced scallions (3)
- Chopped sun-dried tomatoes (.5 c.)
- Ricotta cheese (15 oz.)
- Pepper
- Salt
- Sliced zucchini (3)
- Breakfast polenta (1)
- Olive oil (1 Tbsp.)

Directions:

1. Turn on your oven and let it heat up to 375 degrees. Prepare a baking pan.
2. Make your polenta and then spoon into the prepared pan.
3. Fry some zucchini in a pan with some olive oil until it becomes soft. Place half of the zucchini on top of the polenta.
4. Use a spoon to spread out half the ricotta on the zucchini. Then top this with half the rosemary, Parmesan, mozzarella, garlic, scallions, and tomatoes.
5. Repeat the layers until all ingredients are gone. Place the dish into the oven. After 35 minutes, take it out of the oven. Give it time to rest before serving.

Nutritional Information:

Calories: 356
Fat: 20g
Carbs: 20g
Protein: 28g

White Pizza

Cooking Time: 15 mins
Prep Time: 15 mins

Ingredients:

- Thyme leaves (1 Tbsp.)
- Sliced fennel bulb (.5)
- Sliced leek (1)
- Sliced Fontina cheese (8 oz.)
- Olive oil (1 Tbsp.)
- Salt (1 tsp.)
- Pizza crust, cooked (1)

Directions:

1. Turn the oven on so it can heat up to 400 degrees. Brush some of the oil all over your crust and then you can top with some cheese.
2. Arrange the fennel and leek on top and sprinkle the salt on top. Add it to the oven and let it bake.
3. After ten minutes, take the pizza out of the oven and top with some thyme leaves before serving.

Nutritional Information:

Calories: 393
Fat: 24g
Carbs: 25g

Protein: 33g

Chicken Pizza

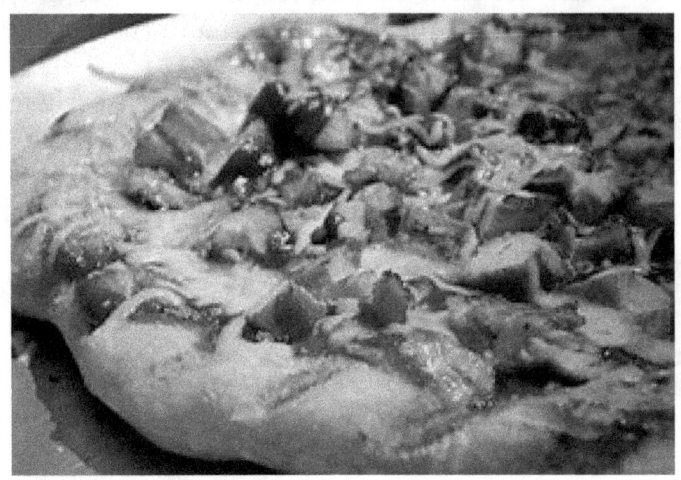

Cooking Time: 15 mins
Prep Time: 15 mins

Ingredients:

- Green olives (.5 c.)
- Parmesan cheese (.5 c.)
- Artichoke hearts (1 can)
- Diced chicken, cooked (2 c.)
- Sliced scallions (3)
- Sliced garlic cloves (2)
- Yogurt cheese (8 oz.)
- Olive oil (1 Tbsp.)
- Cooked pizza crust (1)

Directions:

1. Turn the heat on and let the oven get to 400 degrees. Get the oil prepared and then use it to brush all over the pizza crust.
2. Top the crust with some cheese, garlic, scallions, chicken, artichokes, Parmesan cheese, and olives.
3. Place this into the oven. Cook the pizza until it becomes browned.

Nutritional Information:

Calories: 389
Fat: 13g
Carbs: 30g
Protein: 37g

Linguini Pesto

Cooking Time: 15 mins
Prep Time: 15 mins

Ingredients:

- Parmesan cheese (.5 c.)
- Red pepper slakes (.25 tsp.)
- Sliced olives (.25 c.)
- Baby spinach (2 bags)
- Pesto (.5 c.)
- Olive oil (1 Tbsp.)
- Salt (3 tsp.)
- Linguini (1 lb.)

Directions:

1. Place the noodles in boiling water and cook until it's soft and nice.
2. Add in the red pepper flakes, salt, olives, spinach, pesto, and olive oil. Stir in well.
3. Divide this between a few serving bowls. Top with olive oil and Parmesan cheese.

Nutritional Information:

Calories: 562
Fat: 23g
Carbs: 68g
Protein: 23g

Pasta Primavera

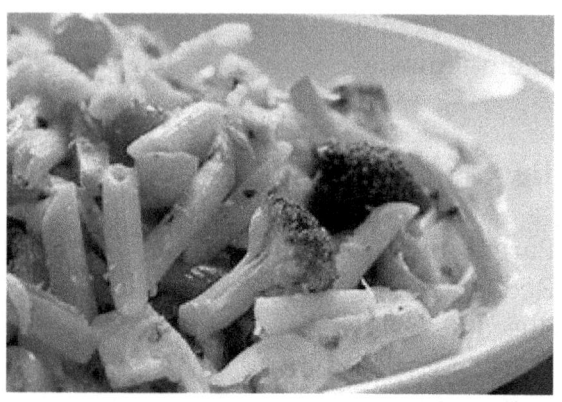

Cooking Time: 15 mins
Prep Time: 15 mins

Ingredients:

- Parmesan cheese (.5 c.)
- Greek yogurt (1 c.)
- Red pepper flakes (.25 tsp.)
- Minced garlic clove (1)
- Sliced carrot (1)
- Peas (1 c.)
- Asparagus (1 bunch)
- Sliced leek (1)
- Olive oil (1 Tbsp.)
- Fettuccini (1 lb.)
- Salt (3 tsp.)

Directions:

1. Boil and prepare the noodles by following the instructions on the package.
2. Bring out a skillet and heat up the oil inside. Cook the leak until they are soft. Add in the red pepper flakes, garlic, some salt, carrot, peas, and asparagus and cook to make them crisp.
3. Place the pasta back into the cooking pot once drained. Add in the cheese, yogurt, and vegetables. Place this into a dish and drizzle with some oil before serving.

Nutritional Information:

Calories: 511
Fat: 10g
Carbs: 80g
Protein: 25g

Shrimp Pasta

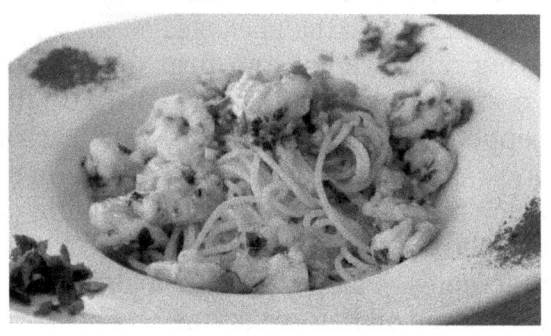

Cooking Time: 15 mins
Prep Time: 15 mins

Ingredients:

- Parmesan cheese (.5 c.)
- Lemon juice (2 Tbsp.)
- Red pepper flakes (.25 tsp.)
- Cooked shrimp (1 lb.)
- Pesto (.5 c.)
- Salt (3 tsp.)

Directions:

1. Cook up the pasta based on the instructions on the box. Drain the water out and return the pasta to the pot.
2. Add in red pepper flakes, lemon juice, shrimp, some salt, and pesto. Mix well until they are thoroughly combined.
3. Place this in a nice dish and top with the Parmesan cheese and olive oil before serving.

Nutritional Information:

Calories: 617
Fat: 20g
Carbs: 65g
Protein: 45g

Vegetarian Dinners for the Mediterranean Diet

Stuffed Tomatoes

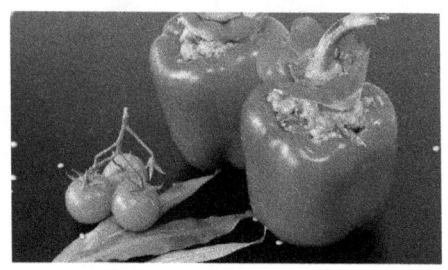

Cooking Time: 30 mins
Prep Time: 20 mins

Ingredients:

- Minced garlic clove (1)
- Pepper
- Dill (1 Tbsp.)
- Olive oil (2 Tbsp. and 1 tsp.)
- Lemon zest (1 Tbsp.)
- Salt
- Sliced scallions (3)
- Chopped kalamata olives (.25 c.)
- Basmati rice (1 c.)
- Water (1.5 c.)
- Tomatoes (4 large)

Directions:

1. Slice the tops off the tomatoes and set aside.
2. Bring out a strainer over a measuring cup. Remove the soft center and the seeds from the tomatoes and let the liquid drain into your measuring cup.
3. Top the tomato liquid with water so you end up with two cups of liquid. Boil the rice, olive oil, water, salt, and tomato in a skillet. Reduce the heat and cook until rice is done.
4. Turn on the oven and heat up to 375 degrees. Spoon the cooked rice into a bowl with the dill, pepper, salt, lemon zest, garlic, scallions, and olives.
5. Add this filling into each tomato and place back its half top. Add to the baking pan and put into the oven.
6. After 15 minutes, take the tomatoes out and enjoy.

Nutritional Information:

Calories: 289
Fat: 10g
Carbs: 47g
Protein: 5g

Fava Beans and Rice

Cooking Time: 20 mins
Prep Time: 10 mins

Ingredients:

- Chopped pistachios (.5 c.)
- Chopped tarragon (1 tsp.)
- Chopped chives (1 Tbsp>0
- Fava beans (1 package)
- Trimmed leek (2)
- Lemon juice (2 Tbsp.)
- Vegetable broth (2.5 c.)
- Salt
- Minced garlic clove (1)
- Olive oil (4 Tbsp.)
- Basmati rice (1 c.)

Directions:

1. Place the broth, salt, garlic, some olive oil, and rice into a pot. Reduce the heat once it boils. Let it cook until the rice becomes soft. Place in the lemon juice and stir.
2. Add the rest of the oil to a skillet. Cook the leeks on it when it's hot before adding some broth and the fava beans. Cook for five minutes.
3. Spoon the rice onto a serving dish and place the vegetables on top. Top with the pistachios, tarragon, and chives.

Nutritional Information:

Calories: 601
Fat: 19g
Carbs: 87g
Protein: 24g

Lebanese Lentils

Cooking Time: 30 mins
Prep Time: 15 mins

Ingredients:

- Lemon (.5)
- Sliced shallots (2)
- Lentils (1 can)
- Water (1.5 c.)
- Cinnamon stick (1)
- Cayenne pepper (.25 tsp.)
- Pepper
- Salt (1 tsp.)
- Cumin seeds (1 tsp.)
- Basmati rice (.75 c.)
- Olive oil (.5 c. and 1 Tbsp.)

Directions:

1. Place some oil in a pot and then add the cumin seeds and rice. Cook five minutes.
2. Add in the water, cinnamon, cayenne, pepper, and salt. Boil all of them in a tightly covered pot. Simmer and cook after boiling until the rice is well-cooked and the water is gone.
3. Stir the lentils into this cooked rice. Add half a cup of oil to a frying pan. When it gets hot, add in the shallots and cook until crispy. Remove with a spoon and drain out the oil.

4. Spoon the rice into a serving platter and top the dish with some shallots. Squeeze lemon on top of it all and serve.

Nutritional Information:

Calories: 574
Fat: 32g
Carbs: 58g
Protein: 15g

Vegetable and Couscous

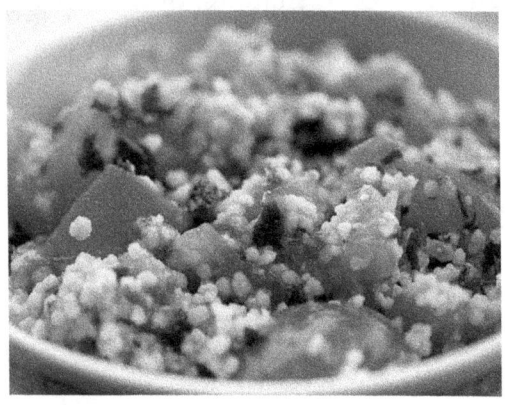

Cooking Time: 25 mins
Prep Time: 15 mins

Ingredients:

- Chopped parsley (.25 c.)
- Minced garlic cloves (1)
- Golden raisins (3 Tbsp.)
- Couscous (2 c.)
- Diced red onion (1)
- Water (3 c.)
- Cayenne pepper (.25 tsp.)
- Salt
- Olive oil (3 Tbsp.)
- Roma tomatoes (4)
- Sliced red bell pepper (1)
- Sliced Brussels sprouts (10)
- Winter squash (3 c.)

Directions:

1. Turn on the oven and let it heat up to 400 degrees. While that warms up, combine the cayenne pepper, salt, oil, tomatoes, garlic, bell pepper, red onion, Brussels sprouts, and winter squash together.
2. Divide these vegetables into two rimmed baking sheets and cover with foil before putting into the oven.
3. After ten minutes, take the foil off and let it cook a bit longer until the vegetables are tender.
4. Place water into a pan and let it boil. Add the couscous and raisins to a bowl and pour the boiling water. Let it sit for a bit.
5. After some time, fluff the couscous and add in some oil, parsley, and salt. Move the couscous over to make a large space in the middle.
6. Spoon the vegetables into the middle and then serve.

Nutritional Information:

Calories: 571
Fat: 12g
Carbs: 103g
Protein: 17g

Mushroom Risotto

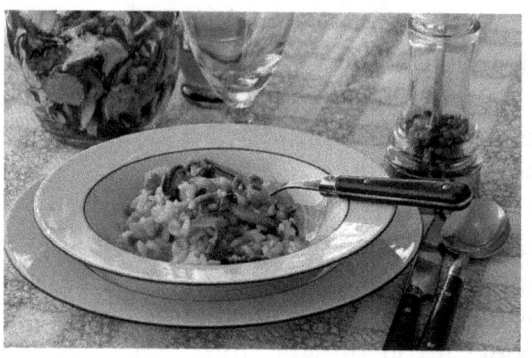

Cooking Time: 25 mins
Prep Time: 15 mins

Ingredients:

- Pepper
- Salt
- Chopped parsley (1 Tbsp.)
- Parmesan cheese (.5 c.)
- Vegetable broth (2 c.)
- Farro (1 c.)
- Red wine (.5 c.)
- Sliced mushrooms (10)
- Sliced shallot (1)
- Olive oil (2 Tbsp.)

Directions:

1. Fry the shallot in a pan with heated oil. Then add in the red wine and mushrooms and let these simmer until the wine evaporates.
2. Add in the farro and half a cup of broth. Let this simmer until the broth evaporates and then repeat until the broth is gone.
3. Turn off the stove heat and add in the parsley, salt, pepper, and cheese. Serve right away.

Nutritional Information:

Calories: 322
Fat: 11g
Carbs: 38g
Protein: 14g

Spinach and Rice Mold

Cooking Time: 50 mins
Prep Time: 15 mins

Ingredients:

- Beaten eggs (2)
- Parmesan cheese (.5 c.)
- Lemon zest (1 Tbsp.)
- Sun-dried tomatoes (.5 c.)
- Water (3.5 c.)
- Pepper
- Salt
- Chopped spinach (1 bag)
- Basmati rice (1.75 c.)
- Diced white onion (1)
- Olive oil (3 Tbsp.)
- Butter (1 Tbsp.)

Directions:

1. Turn on the oven and heat it up to 350 degrees. Prepare a soufflé dish.
2. Brown the onion in some oil in the skillet. Then add in the water, pepper, salt, spinach, and rice and boil these ingredients.
3. Once it boils, let it simmer and ensure the liquid is gone. Spoon this into a bowl and fluff up with a spoon. Let it set a bit.
4. Add in the eggs, cheese, lemon zest, and tomatoes. Spoon this into your soufflé mold

and smooth the top. Cover with some foil and place into a baking pan. Add some water to the larger pan.
5. Add this to the oven and let it bake. After 30 minutes, take the pan out of the oven, get rid of the foil, and serve after slicing.

Nutritional Information:

Calories: 534
Fat: 20g
Carbs: 74g
Protein: 16g

Tunisian Pepper and Eggs

Cooking Time: 15 mins
Prep Time: 10 mins

Ingredients:

- Chopped red bell pepper (1)
- Chopped parsley (2 Tbsp.)
- Minced garlic clove (1)
- Eggs (4)
- Salt
- Water (.5 c.)
- Harissa (1 Tbsp)
- Chopped green bell pepper (1)
- Diced tomatoes (3)
- Cumin seeds (1 tsp.)
- Paprika (1 Tbsp.)
- Sliced onion (1)
- Olive oil (2 Tbsp.)

Directions:

1. Add some oil into a skillet and warm it up before cooking in the cumin seeds, paprika, and onion until toasted.
2. Then add in the salt, water, Harissa, bell peppers, tomatoes, and garlic. Bring this to a simmer and cook to thicken it up.
3. Make four indents into the sauce and crack an egg into each one. Close the pan and cook until the eggs set.

4. Add some parsley to this and then serve.

Nutritional Information:

Calories: 205
Fat: 13g
Carbs: 16g
Protein: 9g

Egyptian Omelet

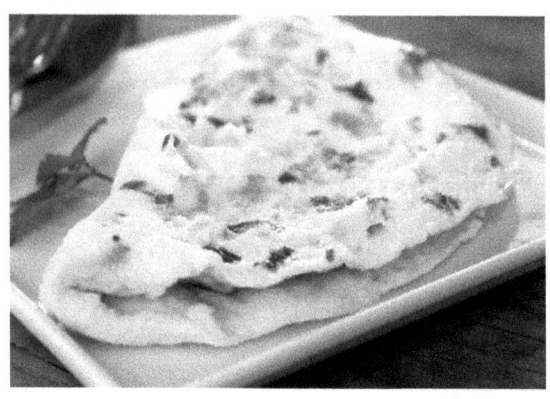

Cooking Time: 20 mins
Prep Time; 10 min

Ingredients:

- Chopped parsley (1 Tbsp.)
- Minced garlic cloves (1)
- Crumbled feta cheese (2 oz.)
- Beaten eggs (8)
- Pepper
- Salt
- Chopped tomatoes (4)
- Chopped onion (1)
- Olive oil (3 Tbsp.)

Directions:

1. Turn on the oven and give it time to heat up to 400 degrees. Warm up some oil in a skillet and then cook the onions to make them soft.
2. Add in the pepper, salt, tomatoes, and garlic and simmer a bit longer.

3. Pour the eggs into this mixture and mix a bit, then let the mixture settle in the bottom.
4. Bake the pan in the oven until the eggs are set.
5. After 5 minutes, take it out of the oven and top with the feta and parsley. Slice up the omelet and serve.

Nutritional Information:

Calories: 295
Fat: 23g
Carbs: 10g
Protein: 15g

Layered Vegetable Casserole

Cooking Time: 45 mins
Prep Time: 30 mins

Ingredients:

- Sliced mozzarella cheese (1 lb.)
- Sliced scallions (2)
- Parmesan cheese (.5 c.)
- Pesto (.5 c.)
- Ricotta cheese (1 lb.)
- Pepper
- Sliced bell peppers (2)
- Salt
- Sliced zucchini (3)
- Sliced eggplant (1)
- Olive oil (3 Tbsp.)

Directions:

1. Turn on the oven and let it heat up to 400 degrees. Prepare a baking pan.
2. Sprinkle some salt over the zucchini and eggplant before placing them on the baking sheet in one layer. Let them stay there for 15 minutes before patting the vegetables dry.
3. In a bowl, combine the olive oil, bell peppers, zucchini, eggplant, pepper, and salt together. On a baking sheet, lay these all in one layer and place into the hot oven.

4. After 10 minutes, take the vegetables out and turn them over. Return so the other side can brown.
5. While that bakes, take out a bowl and combine the scallions, Parmesan, pesto, and ricotta.
6. Place a layer of the vegetables into a pan and top with half the ricotta and some cheese. Repeat the layers until all the ingredients are gone. Turn the temperature of the oven down to 375 degrees.
7. Use a foil to cover the dish and place it into the oven. After 20 minutes, take it out of the oven and let it cool down before eating.

Nutritional Information:

Calories: 420
Fat: 28g
Carbs: 16g
Protein: 29g

Vegetable Stew

Cooking Time: 15 mins
Prep Time: 15 mins

Ingredients:

- Chopped zucchini (2)
- Chopped parsley (.5 c.)
- Black beans (1 can)
- White beans (1 can)
- Chopped garlic cloves (2)
- Dried rosemary
- Pepper
- Salt
- Vegetable broth (4 c.)
- Chopped bell pepper (1)
- Chopped carrot (1)
- Tomatoes, chopped (2)
- Chopped onion (1)
- Olive oil (3 Tbsp.)

Directions:

1. Put a heavy pot on the stove and add the garlic, onion, and oil. Cook to make the onions soft. Add in the carrot, tomatoes, bell pepper, and zucchini and cook for another 3 minutes.
2. Now, add in the rosemary, pepper, salt, and broth and let it boil. Simmer and cook a bit longer.

3. Add in the beans and cook until the beans are heated enough. Ladle this into bowls and garnish with some parsley.

Nutritional Information:

Calories: 504
Fat: 13g
Carbs: 79g
Protein: 26g

Easy Mediterranean Desserts

Lentil Energy Bites

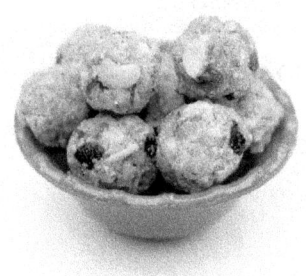

Cooking Time: 30 mins
Prep Time: 40 mins

Ingredients:

- Honey (.5 c.)
- Peanut butter (.5 c.)
- Dark chocolate chips (.25 c.)
- Melted coconut oil (.5 Tbsp.)
- Pumpkin seeds (.25 c.)
- Quick oats, dry (2 c.)
- Shredded coconut (.25 c.)
- Salt
- Coconut flour (1 tsp.)
- Cinnamon (1 tsp.)
- Dry green lentils (.5 c.)

Directions:

1. Turn on the oven and allow it time to heat up to 400 degrees. Use some parchment paper to line up a baking dish.
2. Move the lentils into a pan once it's rinsed. Boil a few cups of water into the pan. Once boiling, lower it a bit and let the lentils simmer for 15 minutes.
3. Drain out the lentils and move to a mixing bowl. Stir in the coconut oil to coat the lentils before sprinkling on the salt, coconut flour, and cinnamon.
4. Spread these lentils onto a baking sheet and add these to the oven. After 15 minutes, stir halfway through and keep checking on them.
5. Take the lentils out of the oven and let them cool down. Combine and stir well the rest of the ingredients with the lentils.
6. Form these into small balls and leave in the refrigerator for 30 minutes to harden before serving.

Nutritional Information:

Calories: 162
Fat: 6.2g
Carbs: 22.6g
Protein: 6g

Black Bean Hummus

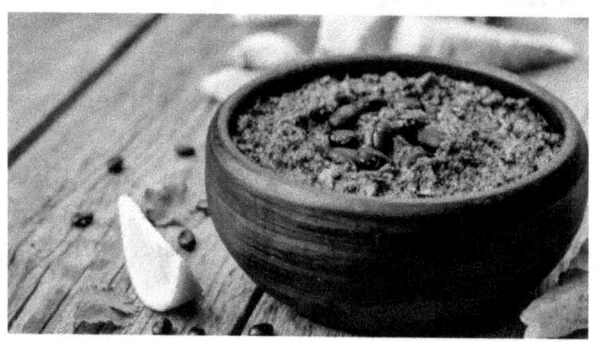

Cooking Time: 0 min
Prep Time: 5 min

Ingredients:

- Olive oil (2 Tbsp.)
- Salt
- Red wine vinegar (3 Tbsp.)
- Sliced garlic cloves (1)
- Almond butter (3 Tbsp.)
- Cottage cheese (2 c.)
- Black beans (2 cans)
- Celery stalks (10)
- Pepper
- Orange zest (2 Tbsp.)
- Parsley (.25 c.)
- Coriander (1 tsp.)
- Cumin (.5 tsp.)

Directions:

1. Bring out your food processor and add in all of your ingredients, besides the celery. Puree this until it is smooth.
2. Move this mixture to a bowl and serve with the celery.

Nutritional Information:

Calories: 218
Fat: 7.5g
Carbs: 20g
Protein: 16g

Roasted Chickpeas

Cooking Time: 30 mins
Prep Time: 25 mins

Ingredients:

- Dried basil (.5 tsp.)
- Garlic powder (.5 tsp.)
- Salt (.25 tsp.)
- Olive oil (1 tsp.)
- Chickpeas (1 can)
- Red pepper flakes (.25 tsp.)
- Nutritional Yeast (1 tsp.)

Directions:

1. Drain out and rinse off the chickpeas, taking the time to pat them dry.
2. Bring out a bowl and combine the oil and chickpeas and mix around. Pour these into a baking sheet that has been covered with foil. Layer them in a single file.
3. Turn on the oven and let it heat up to 450 degrees. Add in the chickpeas and cook for a bit. After 15 minutes, toss around and roast a bit longer.
4. After this time, turn the oven off, open up the oven, and let the chickpeas stay there and cool down for 20 more minutes.
5. Serve when ready.

Nutritional Information:

Calories: 395
Fat: 8.5g
Carbs: 60.5g
Protein: 20.5g

Greek Baklava

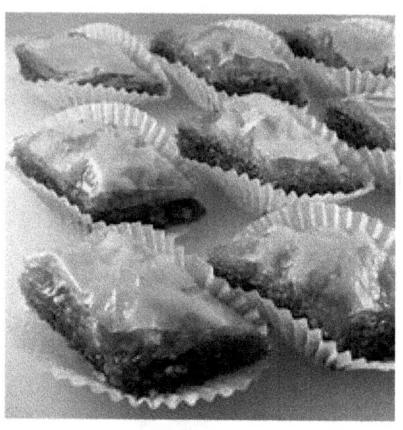

Cooking Time: 50 mins
Prep Time: 15 mins

Ingredients:

- White sugar (1 c.)
- Chopped nuts (1 lb.)
- Phyllo dough (1 package)
- Honey (.5 c.)
- Vanilla (1 tsp.)
- Water (1 c.)
- Cinnamon (1 tsp.)
- Butter (1 c.)

Directions:

1. Turn on the oven and let it heat up to 350 degrees Fahrenheit. Coat the side and bottom of a baking pan with butter.
2. Chop up the nuts before tossing together with the cinnamon. Leave it on one side for awhile.

Take out the phyllo dough and unroll it. Slice the whole stack until it fits the pan. Ensure it doesn't dry out by using a damp cloth.
3. Coat two sheets of dough with butter and place them in a pan. Repeat the layering until you have 8 layers of the sheet in total.
4. Top with the nut mixture. Alternately layer with two sheets of dough, nuts, and butter until the top layer is almost 8 sheets deep.
5. Cut square shapes using a knife to the bottom of the pan. Then bake in the oven.
6. After 50 minutes, you can take it out. While that is baking, work on the sauce. Boil the water and sugar together to melt the sugar. Then add the vanilla and honey and simmer for 20 minutes.
7. Remove the baklava and then spoon the sauce on top. Let it cool and then serve.

Nutritional Information:

Calories: 393
Fat: 26g
Carbs: 37g
Protein: 6g

Pumpkin Pie Smoothie

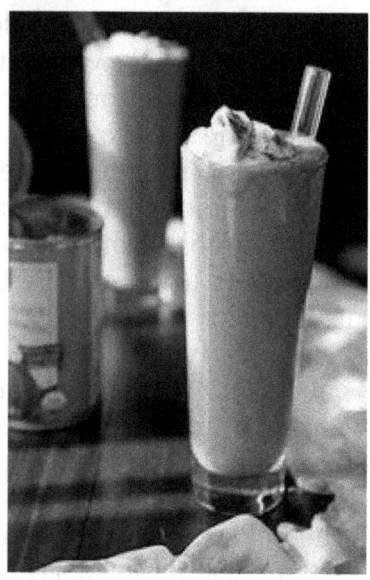

Cooking Time: 0 mins
Prep Time: 5 mins

Ingredients:

- Ground ginger (1 pinch)
- Cinnamon (.25 tsp.)
- Pumpkin puree (.25 c.)
- Yogurt (.25 c.)
- Banana (1)
- Ice cubes (8)

Directions:

1. Take outa blender and blend together the ginger, cinnamon, pumpkin, yogurt, banana, and ice cubes.
2. When these are smooth, pour out into a glass and enjoy.

Nutritional Information:

Calories: 84
Fat: 0.8g
Carbs: 18.6g
Protein: 2.6g

Key Lime Pie

Cooking Time: 0 mins
Prep Time: 5 mins

Ingredients:

- Whipped topping (8 oz.)
- Boiling water (.25 c.)
- Lime gelatin, sugar-free (1 package)
- Key lime pie yogurt (2 boxes)
- Graham cracker crust (1)

Directions:

1. Take out a bowl and let the gelatin dissolve in some boiling water.
2. When the gelatin is dissolved, whisk the yogurt with a wire whisk.
3. Use a wooden spoon to fold in the whipped. Spread this mixture into the crust.
4. Chill for at least 2 hours.

Nutritional Information:

Calories: 43
Fat: 1.4g
Carbs: 7.1g
Protein: 1g

Chocolate Cupcakes

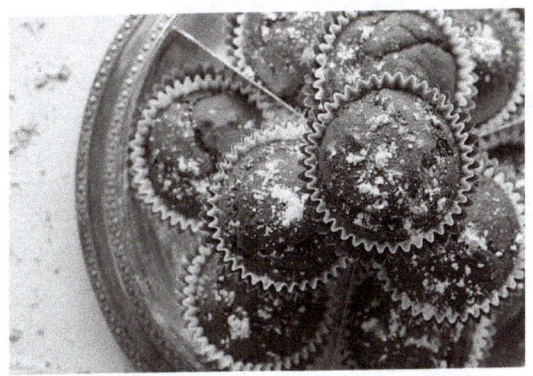

Prep Time: 10 mins
Cooking Time: 35 mins

Ingredients:

- Water (.5 c.)
- Devil's food cake mix (18 oz.)
- Pumpkin (1 can)

Directions:

1. Turn on the oven and allow it to heat up to 350 degrees.
2. Bring out a bowl and mix all the ingredients together by hand or using a mixer.
3. Pour the mixture into some mini muffin tins. When they are full, place into the oven and bake.
4. After 30 minutes, take the cupcakes out and let them cool down before serving.

Nutritional Information:

Calories: 127.7
Fat: 4.5g
Carbs: 22.3g
Protein: 2g

Frozen Pie

Cooking Time: 0 min
Prep Time: 5 mins

Ingredients:

- Light yogurt (6 oz.)
- Cool whip (1 container)

Directions:

1. Take both of these ingredients and mix them together well.
2. Pour into a plain pie plate, or into a crust of your choice, spread out well.
3. After this is done, place the pie into the freezer and wait until it sets before enjoying.

Nutritional Information:

Calories: 12.1
Fat: 1g
Carbs: 1g
Protein: 0.7g

Apple Caramel Fluff

Cooking Time: 0 min
Prep Time: 5 mins

Ingredients:

- Cool Whip (12 oz.)
- Chopped apples (4)
- Crushed pineapple (8 oz.)
- Butterscotch pudding (1 oz.)

Directions:

1. Take out a bowl and mix together the pineapple and the dry pudding.
2. When those two ingredients are well combined, add in the cool whip and the apples.
3. Place this bowl into the fridge and let it sit for a few hours before you serve.

Nutritional Information:

Calories: 51.5
Fat: .1g
Carbs: 13.6g
Protein: 0.3g

Pumpkin Cupcakes

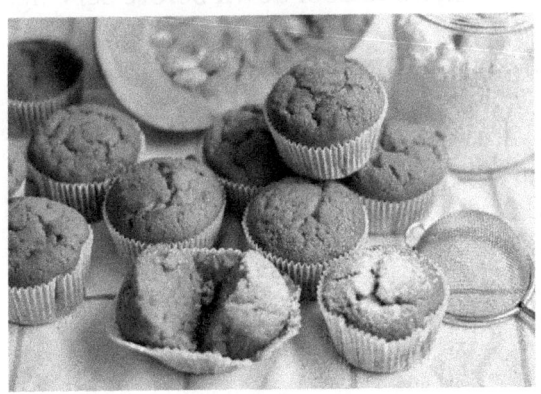

Cooking Time: 25 mins
Prep Time: 10 mins

Ingredients:

- Cinnamon (1.5 tsp.)
- Vanilla (1 tsp.)
- Canned pumpkin (15 oz.)
- Water (1 c.)
- Spice cake mix (1 box)

Directions:

1. Turn on the oven and give it time to heat up to 350 degrees. Prepare a cupcake pan with some liners.
2. Bring out a bowl and combine together the spice cake mix, water, canned pumpkin, vanilla, and cinnamon.
3. Pour the mixture into your prepared cupcake pan and place the whole thing into the oven.

4. Take them out of the oven after 25 minutes and allow them to cool down before serving.

Nutritional Information:

Calories: 100
Fat: 3g
Carbs: 17.5g
Protein: 1.1g

Almonds with Apricots

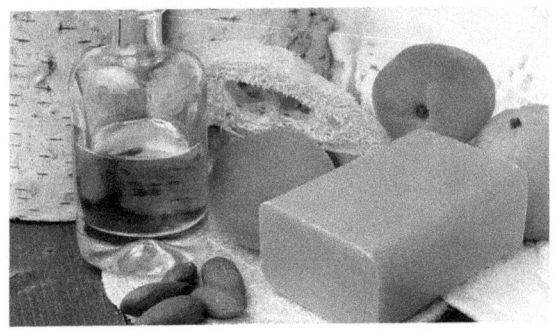

Cooking Time: 5 mins
Prep Time: 10 mins

Ingredients:

- Chopped apricots (.5 c.)
- Cinnamon
- Red pepper flakes
- Salt
- Almonds (1 c.)
- Olive oil (2 Tbsp.)

Directions:

1. Bring out a skillet and add the salt, almonds, and olive oil. Fry for 10 minutes, stirring the whole time.
2. Spoon the almonds into a dish and add the apricot pieces, cinnamon, and red pepper flakes.
3. Cool down before serving.

Nutritional Information:

Calories: 207
Fat: 19g
Carbs: 7g
Protein: 5g

Melon Granita

Prep Time: 10 mins
Freezing Time: 3 hours

Ingredients:

- Chopped mint (2 tsp.)
- Lemon juice (1 Tbsp.)
- Honeydew (1)
- Water (.5 c.)
- Sugar (.5 c.)

Directions:

1. Take out a pan and heat up the water and sugar. Stir to dissolve the sugar and then cool down completely.
2. When the sugar is cool, place into a blender along with the mint, lemon juice, and melon. Blend together well.
3. Pour into a freezer-safe dish and put into the freezer.
4. After an hour, break up the mixture using a fork. Do this every 30 minutes for the next few hours.
5. Spoon into some serving dishes and serve.

Nutritional Information:

Calories: 211
Fat: 0g

Carbs: 54g
Protein: 1g

Balsamic Figs

Cooking Time: 15 mins
Prep Time: 15 mins

Ingredients:

- Almond biscotti (.5 c.)
- Chevre (.5 lb.)
- Salt
- Butter (2 Tbsp.)
- Rosemary (4 sprigs)
- Cinnamon (.5 tsp.)
- Balsamic vinegar (1 Tbsp.)
- Honey (.5 c.)
- Figs (12)
- Olive oil (1 Tbsp.)

Directions:

1. Heat up the oven to 375 degrees. Bring out a bowl and combine the salt, rosemary, cinnamon, vinegar, honey, oil, and butter. Pour this into a baking dish.
2. Add to the oven and let the figs bake. After ten minutes, take out of the oven. Slice the chevre into four pieces and place one piece in each dish.
3. Pour the roasted fruit on top and garnish with some of the biscotti that has been crushed.

Nutritional Information:

Calories: 532
Fat: 23g
Carbs: 77g
Protein: 14g

Yogurt Cheese and Berries

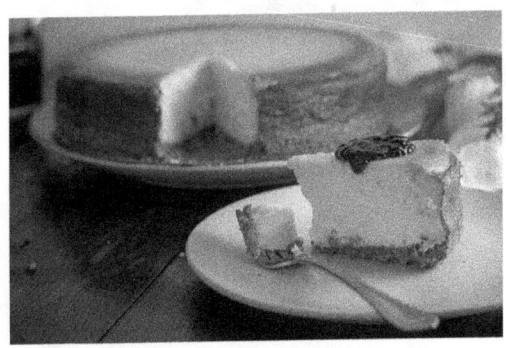

Prep Time: 15 minutes

Ingredients:

- Almonds (.25 c.)
- Balsamic vinegar (1 Tbsp.)
- Honey (3 Tbsp.)
- Berries (3 c.)
- Plain yogurt (6 c.)

Directions:

1. Line cheesecloth into a mesh strainer and then spoon the yogurt inside. Fold the cheesecloth over the yogurt and put over a bowl. Refrigerate overnight.
2. The next day, invert the yogurt cheese onto a plate.
3. Take out a bowl and mix the balsamic vinegar, honey, and berries. Mash the berries up a bit.
4. Spoon this over the yogurt cheese and top with the almonds.

Nutritional Information:

Calories: 379
Fat: 8g
Carbs: 48g
Protein: 23g

Date Night Parfait

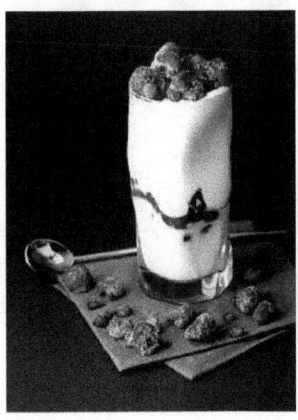

Prep Time: 15 mins

Ingredients:

- Cinnamon (1 tsp.)
- Honey (.5 c.)
- Chopped walnuts (.5 c.)
- Chopped dates (8)
- Greek yogurt (4 c.)

Directions:

1. Place a bit of yogurt at the bottom of four glasses.
2. Top with a layer of dates, some walnuts, and honey. Add in another layer of yogurt and repeat the layering.
3. Dust with some cinnamon and then serve.

Nutritional Information:

Calories: 448
Fat: 12g
Carbs: 67g
Protein: 18g

Apricot Cake

Cooking Time: 35 mins
Prep Time: 15 mins

Ingredients:

- Apricot halves (1 package)
- Vanilla (2 tsp.)
- Rice flour (2 Tbsp.)
- Chopped walnuts (1.25 c.)
- Sugar (1 c.(
- Eggs (3)
- Olive oil (.33 c.)

Directions:

1. Turn on the oven and heat it up to 375 degrees. Prepare a pie plate with some oil.
2. Blend together the vanilla, rice flour, walnuts, sugar, eggs, and oil. Process to make smooth.
3. Arrange the apricots into your pie plate and pour the batter on top. Put into the oven.
4. After 35 minutes, take the cake out and cool before serving.

Nutritional Information:

Calories: 442
Fat: 29g
Carbs: 42g
Protein: 10g

Cherry Clafoutis

Cooking Time: 35 mins
Prep Time: 10 mins

Ingredients:

- Pitted cherries (3 c.)
- Salt
- All-purpose flour (.5 c.)
- Vanilla (1 Tbsp.)
- Eggs (2)
- Sugar (.5 c.)
- Milk (1.25 c.)
- Almonds (.5 c.)
- Butter (2 Tbsp.)

Directions:

1. Turn on the oven and allow it to heat up to 350 degrees. Prepare a pie plate with some butter and add the ground almonds.
2. Add the vanilla, salt, flour, eggs, milk, and half the sugar into the blender. Process until smooth. Pour the mixture into the pie plate and arrange the cherries on top with the sugar.
3. Bake in the oven. After 35 minutes, take out of the oven and cool before serving.

Nutritional Information:

Calories: 407
Fat: 16g
Carbs: 57g
Protein: 10g

Chocolate Brownies

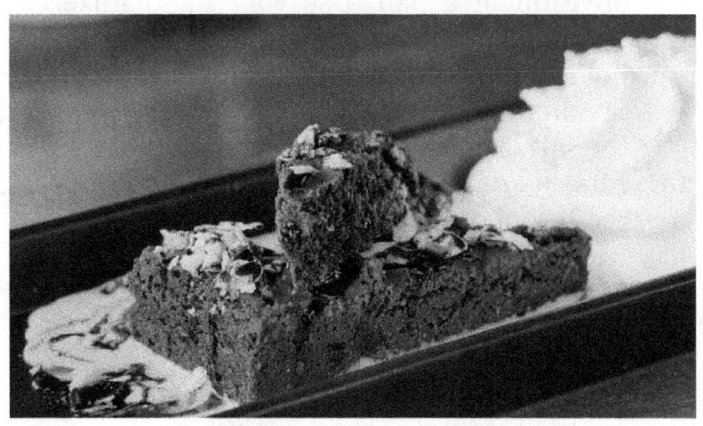

Cooking Time: 35 mins
Prep Time: 15 mins

Ingredients:

- Salt
- Cocoa (.25 c.)
- All-purpose flour (.5 c.)
- Melted bittersweet chocolate (8 oz.)
- Vanilla (2 tsp.)
- Egg (1)
- Sugar (.75 c.)
- Olive oil (.25 c.)

Directions:

1. Turn on the oven and let it heat up to 375 degrees. Prepare a pan.

2. Combine together the vanilla, egg, sugar, and olive oil in a pan. Use your hand mixer and beat it until light and fluffy.
3. Fold in the cocoa powder, flour, and chocolate. Spoon this into your prepared pan and sprinkle the salt on top before adding to the oven.
4. After 35 minutes, take the brownies out and let them cool down before slicing.

Nutritional Information:

Calories: 214
Fat: 11g
Carbs: 29g
Protein: 3g

Easy Smoothies for Those Busy Days

Walnut Smoothie

Prep Time: 10 mins

Ingredients:

- Ice
- Vanilla (.5 tsp.)
- Cinnamon (.5 tsp.)
- Walnuts (.33 c.)
- Milk (.5 c.)
- Pitted dates (4)
- Plain Greek yogurt (2 c.)

Directions:

1. Take out your blender and combine the ice, vanilla, cinnamon, walnuts, milk, dates, and yogurt.
2. Blend these until they are nice and smooth.
3. Pour into two glasses and serve.

Nutritional Information:

Calories: 384
Fat: 17g
Carbs: 35g
Protein: 21g

Turmeric Smoothie

Prep Time: 10 mins

Ingredients:

- Ice
- Ground turmeric (.5 tsp.)
- Honey (3 Tbsp>)
- Cored green apple (.5)
- Fennel bulb (.5)
- Orange juice (1 c.)
- Carrot juice (2 c.)

Directions:

1. Bring out a blender and combine the ice, turmeric, honey, apple, fennel, orange juice, and carrot juice.
2. When this is nice and smooth, pour into two glasses and serve.

Nutritional Information:

Calories: 241
Fat: 1g
Carbs: 61g
Protein: 3g

Minty Smoothie

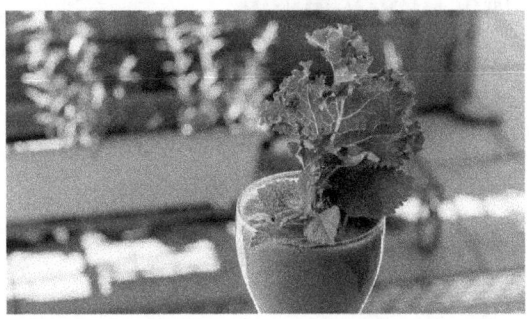

Prep Time: 15 mins

Ingredients:

- Lemon juice (1 Tbsp.)
- Ice
- Chopped mint (2 Tbsp)
- Salt
- Sugar (1 tsp.)
- Olive oil (1 Tbsp.)
- Ripe tomato (1)
- Sliced cucumber (1)

Directions:

1. Take out the blender and add all of the ingredients inside. Put the lid on top of the blender.
2. Blend the ingredients together until they are smooth.
3. Pour into two glasses and then serve right away.

Nutritional Information:

Calories: 100
Fat: 7g
Carbs: 9g
Protein: 2g

Lassi

Prep Time: 10 mins

Ingredients:

- Ice (1 c.)
- Saffron threads
- Rosewater (2 tsp.)
- Sugar (.5 c.)
- Milk (1.5 c.)
- Plain yogurt (2 c.)

Directions:

1. Bring out a blender and combine the saffron, rose water, ice, sugar, milk, and yogurt.
2. Blend these until they are smooth.
3. Serve in four glasses.

Nutritional Information:

Calories: 227
Fat: 3g
Carbs: 38g
Protein: 10g

Early Morning Frappe

Prep Time: 10 mins

- Ice
- Turkish coffee (1 Tbsp.)
- Maple syrup (.25 c.)
- Almond milk (2.5 c.)

Directions:

1. Take out your blender and combine the ice, coffee, maple syrup, and almond milk.
2. Blend these until they are nice and smooth.
3. Pour the mixture into two glasses before serving.

Nutritional Information:

Calories: 153
Fat: 5g
Carbs: 29g
Protein: 1g

Chamomile Tea

Prep Time: 10 mins

Ingredients:

- Ice cubes
- Lemon peel (4 strips)
- Boiling water (4 c.)
- Honey (.25 c.)
- Lemon juice (.25 c.)
- Chamomile tea (4 bags)

Directions:

1. Bring out your teapot and place the honey, lemon, and chamomile inside. Pour some boiling water on top of these ingredients and let them steep.
2. After five minutes, take the tea bags out of the pot and pour this into a pitcher. Let it chill.
3. When it is time to serve, twist strips of the lemon peel to get the oils into each glass. Add the ice and serve.

Nutritional Information:

Calories: 68
Fat: 0g
Carbs: 18g
Protein: 0g

Raspberry Fizz

Prep Time: 10 mins

Ingredients:

- Chilled Prosecco (1 bottle)
- Chopped mint (2 tsp.)
- Lemon juice (1 Tbsp.)
- Raspberry jam (2 Tbsp.)
- Raspberries (1 pint)

Directions:

1. Place the lemon juice, raspberry jam, and berries into a bowl. Mash the berries to release the juices.
2. Place some of these berries into each glass along with some of the chopped mint.
3. Slowly add in the Prosecco so as not to overflow. Stir once before serving.

Nutritional Information:

Calories: 204
Fat: 1g
Carbs: 18g
Protein: 1g

30-Day Meal Plan to Get You Started

Day: 1	Day: 2	Day : 3	Day: 4	Day: 5
Breakfast: Scrambled Eggs Lunch: Tuna Patties Dinner: Easy Tuna Salad Snack: Lentil Energy Bites	Breakfast: Egg Salad Lunch: Pasta and Smoked Salmon Dinner: Grilled Salmon Kebabs Snack: Black Bean Hummus	Breakfast: Sunny Quinoa Breakfast Bowl Lunch: Salmon Quinoa Burgers Dinner: Cilantro Tilapia Snack: Roasted Chickpeas	Breakfast: Honey Caramelized Figs Lunch: Chicken and Rice Soup Dinner: Shrimp Skewers Snack: Greek Baklava	Breakfast: Mediterranean Toast Lunch: Tuna and Egg Salad Dinner: Chicken with Mushrooms
Day: 6	Day: 7	Day: 8	Day: 9	Day: 10
Breakfast: Mediterranean Potato Hash	Breakfast: Breakfast Egg Muffins	Breakfast: Breakfast Tostadas	Breakfast: Classic Mediterranean Breakfas	Breakfast: Veggie Quiche Lunch:

Lunch: Fennel and Crab Salad Dinner: Tomato and Chicken Salad Snack: Pumpkin Pie Smoothie	Lunch: Zucchini Panini Dinner: Lemony Chicken Snack: Key Lime Pie	Lunch: Greek Village Salad Dinner: Chicken Rollatini Snack: Chocolate Cupcakes	t Lunch Chicken Corn Salad: Dinner: Turkey Burgers Snack: Frozen Pie	Chicken Fried Rice Dinner: Mussels with Garlic and Wine Snack: Apple Caramel Fluff
Day: 11 Breakfast: Mediterranean Omelet Lunch: Turkey Tacos Dinner: Shrimp Scampi Snack: Pumpkin	Day: 12 Breakfast: Mediterranean Breakfast Salad Lunch: Asparagus and Pork Dinner: Chicken Cacciatore	Day: 13 Breakfast: Greek-Style Frittata Lunch: Pork Chops Dinner: Stuffed Chicken Snack: Almond	Day: 14 Breakfast: Kale and Goat Cheese Frittata Lunch: Chicken Tostados Dinner: Pork Loin Snack:	Day: 15 Breakfast: Greek Vegetable and Feta Cheese Pie Lunch: Caprese Wrap Dinner: Lamb Meatball

| Cupcakes | Snack: Chocolate Cupcakes | s with Apricots | Melon Granita | s

Snack: Balsamic Figs |
|---|---|---|---|---|
| Day: 16

Breakfast: Breakfast Sandwiches

Lunch: Aram Sandwich

Dinner: Pomegranate Lamb Shanks

Snack: Yogurt Cheese and Berries | Day: 17

Breakfast: Fava Beans with Pita Bread

Lunch: Grilled Veggie Wrap

Dinner: Polenta Lasagna

Snack: Date Night Parfait | Day: 18

Breakfast: Yogurt and Honey Fruit Delight

Lunch: Tomato and Feta Ciabatta

Dinner: White Pizza

Snack: Apricot Cake | Day: 19

Breakfast: Apricot Muesli

Lunch: Tuscan Tuna Pita

Dinner: Chicken Pizza

Snack: Cherry Clafoutis | Day: 20

Breakfast: Breakfast Polenta

Lunch: Lamb Mint Sliders

Dinner: Linguini Pesto

Snack: Chocolate Brownies |
| Day: 21

Breakfast: | Day: 22

Breakfast: | Day: 23

Breakfast: | Day: 24

Breakfast: | Day: 25

Breakfast: |

Zucchini Muffins Lunch: Mushroom Pesto Pizza Dinner: Pasta Primavera Snack: Walnut Smoothie	Baked Eggs Lunch: Fava Beans with Pita Bread Dinner: Shrimp Pasta Snack: Turmeric Smoothie	Feta Frittata Lunch: Pork Chops Dinner: Polenta Lasagna Snack: Minty Smoothie	Batsaria Lunch: Caprese Wrap Dinner: Chicken Pizza Snack: Chocolate Brownies	Scrambled Eggs Lunch: Chicken Tostados Dinner: White pizza Snack: Lassi
Day: 26 Breakfast: Mediterranean Breakfast Salad Lunch: Tuscan Tuna Pita Dinner: Lamb meatballs	Day: 27 Breakfast: Breakfast Sandwiches Lunch: Lamb Mint Sliders Dinner: Shrimp Scampi	Day: 28 Breakfast: Greek Style Frittata Lunch: Asparagus and Pork Dinner: Pomegranate Lamb	Day: 29 Breakfast: Yogurt and Honey Fruit Delight Lunch: Pork Chops Dinner: Turkey Burgers	Day: 30 Breakfast: Zucchini Muffins Lunch: Turkey Tacos Dinner: Cilantro Tilapia Snack: Raspberry Fizz

| Snack: Pumpkin Cupcakes | Snack: Early Morning Frappe | Shanks

Snack: Chamomile Tea | Snack: Date Night Parfait | |

Conclusion

Congratulations, you've reached the end of the book! I hope these habits last you a lifetime and your relationship with food will be revolutionized forever. If this book has helped you in any way please leave us a review, it would mean a lot!

Thank you for reading!

www.ingramcontent.com/pod-product-compliance
Lightning Source LLC
Chambersburg PA
CBHW051541020426